What Others Are Saying About This Book

Dr. Bob DeMaria's book, Dr. Bob's Drugless Guide to Balance Female Hormones *, is a must read for every woman. Being a woman is not easy: There are hot flashes, mood swings and fatigue, along with pressures and the stress of daily life. Through concise, easy-to-read chapters that explain what our bodies are really going through, Dr. Bob walks you through practical solutions to feeling better through diet, exercise, and natural supplements. We cannot always change our circumstances— but we can change our body so that we are not overwhelmed by day-to-day challenges. This book helps you make lifestyle changes for a healthier, happier life.*
~Marilyn Hickey
President and Founder of Marilyn Hickey Ministries

As a Women's Health & Fertility Naturopathic Specialist, this book is now on my MUST READ list for every patient that comes into my practice. It is so vital to understand the truth about women's hormones. More so, it's important to appreciate the subtle dance of hormonal interrelationships and how powerful natural medicines, whole-food diet and stress management help to create hormonal balance for the rest of a woman's life! The realistic, achievable and powerful hormone-balancing strategies Dr. Bob will teach you in this book, will guide you to achieve the results you've dreamed of—drug-free, optimal, hormonal health!
~Dr. Angela Hywood ND
Holistic Gynecological, Obstetrical & Natural Fertility Specialist

Dr. DeMaria makes a valuable contribution to the often confusing, always vital battle of bringing balance to female hormones. Add this book to your library!
~David J. Fraham, ND,
President and Founder, Health Quarters Ministries

As a 39-year-old mother of three small children, I was experiencing problems common to many women of my age. My migraines, most notably, were being poorly treated by conventional healthcare, and they were getting worse.

Following Dr. Bob's advice, many of my symptoms have dramatically improved or resolved. After three months, I look better and feel younger. I am a true believer in Dr. Bob's approach to healing from the inside out. **~P. Brethauer, MD**

Dr. Bob's Drugless Guide To Balance Female Hormones

BY
Drugless Healthcare Solutions
Dr. Robert F. DeMaria

Dr. Bob's Drugless Guide to Balance Female Hormones
by Robert DeMaria, D.C.

Published by:
Drugless Healthcare Solutions
P.O. Box 136
Avon, OH 44011

Phone:	(440) 323-3841
Fax:	(440) 322-2502
E-Mail:	druglesscare@aol.com
Web site:	www.DruglessDoctor.com

Library of Congress Control Number: 2007906534
ISBN: 978-0-9728907-3-1

Printed in the United States of America
0 9 8 7 6 5 4 3 2 1

DISCLAIMER

Book cover design by www.Newbomb.com
Page design by One-On-One Book Production, West Hills, CA

About Dr. Bob

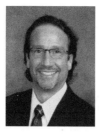

Dr. Bob has been helping patients with natural drugless care since the 1970s. Over his career he has noticed a progressive decline in the quality of life that new patients present to his office. What used to occur in individuals, especially females who were fifty and sixty, is now happening to women in their thirties and forties. The magnitude of surgeries and invasive procedures has escalated to the point where nearly every new patient, young or old, has been prescribed a medication or has experienced some type of surgical intervention. These facts have motivated him to pursue finding natural drugless answers for conditions that are occurring in epidemic proportions and continuing at an alarming rate. Hundreds of thousands of hysterectomies, cholecystectomies (gallbladder extraction), and breast cyst removal can be prevented by making appropriate lifestyle modifications.

Dr. Bob has a Bachelors degree in Human Biology. He is a practicing DC and has relentlessly continued with his post graduate education, earning a Natural Health Doctor degree (NHD), a Fellow status in Spinal Engineering and Diplomat status in treating bone and joint conditions without medication. Dr. Bob graduated Valedictorian of his class with honors. He is a recognized world-wide expert and frequently is a keynote speaker.

He teaches post-graduate level, continuing education classes in the health, business, legal and teaching professions. Doctor Bob has been a College instructor, and has spoken in Europe and Canada. He has been on TV internationally, and he hosts his own weekly regional TV program with his wife of over thirty years, Deb. He has two sons.

Dr. Bob has three popular selling books focusing on health restoration naturally; including *"Dr. Bob's Guide to Stop ADHD in 18 Days," "Dr. Bob's Trans Fat Survival Guide"* and *"Dr. Bob's Guide to Optimal Health." "Dr. Bob's Guide to Balancing Female Hormones"* is an accumulation of thirty plus years of experience that will surely make a difference in anyone's life.

Dr. Bob knows it is time for the public to take control of their own future in reference to the state of their personal health. He knows it can work, he sees it happen everyday. The information in this book will make a difference. All you have to do, is take action. Today is your day.

Acknowledgments

The information that you will find in this book is an integral part of my clinical career. Female patients have suffered much over the years with strong prescriptions that have altered a generation with serious side effects. Recently, there was a government-sponsored study that was tracking the effects of hormone replacement therapy. After revealing that hormone replacement therapy may cause heart disease and other blood vessel challenges, the study was brought to an abrupt halt. This was very positive because quick action has saved thousands of lives.

I would like to acknowledge my female patients who have made appropriate lifestyle changes resulting in a healthy hormone life. Congratulations to each of you who continue to pursue optimal health naturally in spite of all the pressures of the medical community to take prescription medication.

Thank you to the editors and readers of the manuscript: Teri Forthofer, Laura Meyer, Dr. Jack Kohl and my typist and liaison editor, Kim Plaso. I would like to thank Connie Schnorr and Sue Dowden who helped with the final details. Chantelle Layton for her artistic assistance and Karen Hurguy, whose drawings were used to depict the functions of the body. A special expression of gratitude to my friend and colleague, Dr. John Madeira, for sharing his familiarity and insight into the Amish community and their lifestyle.

I would not be in a position to create the several books I have been able to generate without the unconditional support and passion from my wife, Deb. She has been a consistent motivator, knowing that we are making an impact on our generation. I would also like to thank my sons, Dominic and Anthony, who have been a joy to raise and have seen how natural healthcare can make a difference.

I would like to acknowledge all of you, the readers, who have an opportunity to improve your health without medication. Congratulations in advance as you explore the new realm of optimal health; I promise, you will not be disappointed.

Dr. Bob

TABLE OF CONTENTS

PREFACE · xi

INTRODUCTION · 1

PART I —
TEN NATURAL POINTS TO OPTIMAL FEMALE HEALTH

CHAPTER ONE: **Hormones:** The Basics · · · · · · · · · · · **11**

CHAPTER TWO: **Estrogen** and the Liver · · · · · · · · · · **29**

CHAPTER THREE: **Progesterone** · · · · · · · · · · · · · **43**

CHAPTER FOUR: Other **Hormones** Affecting the Balance · · · **53**

CHAPTER FIVE: Let's Talk About the **Lymphatic System** · · · **57**

CHAPTER SIX: Importance of Optimal **Liver** Function · · · · **67**

CHAPTER SEVEN: Fuel the **Thyroid** to Keep the Body Going **77**

CHAPTER EIGHT: Supporting the **Adrenal Glands** · · · · · · **89**

CHAPTER NINE: Strengthen the **Frame** and **Structure** · · · **101**

CHAPTER TEN: **Communication** Between the Brain and
Tissue Cells · **121**

PART II —
LEARN HOW TO WAKE UP THE DETECTIVE INSIDE OF YOU

CHAPTER ELEVEN: **Common Female Conditions** That are
Challenging · **133**

CHAPTER TWELVE: What Causes **Hot Flashes?** · · · · · · · **141**

CHAPTER THIRTEEN: Learning From the **Amish** · · · · · · · **155**

PART III —
JUST TELL ME WHAT TO DO

CHAPTER FOURTEEN: How Do You **Exercise?** · · · · · · · · **165**

CHAPTER FIFTEEN: What **Tests** Should You Have
Completed? · **171**

CHAPTER SIXTEEN: Reversing Unhealthy Patterns · · · · · **189**

CHAPTER SEVENTEEN: Cleansing Protocols · · · · · · · · **201**

CHAPTER EIGHTEEN: What Supplements Do You Need? · · **219**

CHAPTER NINETEEN: How to Get Off Your **Medication** · · · **225**

PART IV —
YOU ARE WHAT YOU EAT

CHAPTER TWENTY: **The Page Fundamental Diet Plan** · · · **233**

CHAPTER TWENTY-ONE: **Food Transition Guide —**
Steps to Change · **247**

CHAPTER TWENTY-TWO: **FACTS** About **FAT** · · · · · · · · **251**

CHAPTER TWENTY-THREE: **Sweet Alternatives** and the
Glycemic Index · **271**

CHAPTER TWENTY-FOUR: Acquiring Your **Normal Weight**
Naturally! · **283**

PART V — CONCLUDING THOUGHTS

CHAPTER TWENTY-FIVE: **Finishing the Puzzle** · · · · · · · **299**

CHAPTER TWENTY-SIX: Bonus Chapter: Balancing **Male**
Hormones · **303**

CONCLUDING THOUGHTS · · · · · · · · · · · · · · · · · **311**

APPENDIX · **313**

INDEX · **335**

Preface

Congratulation on choosing this Natural Health Guide that has the potential to positively impact you and your family's lives for generations to come. We are living in a time of great knowledge and awesome technological advances. It appears, as you look from the outside in, that if you have any type of condition where your body is not functioning properly all you have to do is go to your healthcare provider and you will be prescribed a pill, potion or cream and everything will be better. When you read magazines and news articles today you are led to believe the healthcare industry has a handle on all situations involving sickness.

Investigation and experimentation are being conducted on a variety of very new ideas including stem-cell research and gene pooling. We have successfully used artificial organs and human organ transplants that lengthen the lives of many who faced premature death. I would like to applaud all the very fine physicians and scientists who passionately do their very best to help satisfy the desire of the public—to find answers to these very elusive questions and concerns.

The real truth of the matter is, as a general mass of human flesh, we are not as healthy as it is being portrayed on television and in news releases. It was recently reported, with the intention of reassuring us that the research dollars are helpful and used wisely, that there were a few thousand less deaths from cancer over the last couple of years.

Another publication released a statement that the amount of cancer has diminished in the last couple of years, not because of new procedures, but from the fact that women have made a choice on their own to reduce the amount of hormone replacement therapy they are taking. Conflicting information? Yes. Are we getting the truth from the scientific circles? One of the commentators in the article suggested that even though people may be surviving the aggression of cancer, their post cancer treatment has left them disfigured. I would also like to point out that while patients may live a season longer with a transplanted organ, they are also suffering with the side effects of anti-rejection drugs.

Considering that billions of dollars have been spent over the last several decades one might think that the cancer statistics would be constantly on a downward spiral. I would like to suggest that if we have the technology to increase gas mileage in a vehicle and send operational equipment to Mars, surely it's logical we should be able to solve some of the common ailments that appear to be increasing in intensity and destruction.

A sobering thought, especially with the very positive statistics from the reduction of synthetic hormone replacement correlated with reduced cancers. Is the right treatment approach being pursued for female health? The government has had to step in and suggest that the years of hormone replacement therapy may be causing more harm than good. Recently, it was released that hormone replacement therapy may be safe for select age groups. It is very frustrating as a consumer to know what information you can really trust. How much is motivated by profit? We are talking about the lives of individuals, not patty cake kid games.

Recently, the media has been inundating us with articles that would make one think we are waiting for a flu epidemic to wipe out humanity. There are daily news releases of potentially disastrous ailments lurking to attack you and create total misery in you and your family's lives. I would like to tell you that it is not all that bleak. I also want to be one of the first to tell you that you do have control over your current and future health. The body functions at the cellular level. That means if you feed the body real, whole food, hydrate it with pure water, exercise it on a consistent basis, give it time to have an opportunity to rest and restore function, maintain the spinal structure that connects the brain to the tissue cell, enabling proper nervous system function, you will get well and stay well.

"But, Dr. Bob, I have not felt good my whole life; can you still help me?" is a common statement I hear regularly in my practice; "I have had my gallbladder, colon and uterus removed." The logical answer I commonly respond with is, "I have good news and I have bad news. The good news is, we can support the function you have and improve it by educating you to make logical, healthy life choices. The bad news is, we cannot reverse the loss of the organ."

Often, the patient expects normal function can be restored after an organ has been removed, and this is a challenge to the healthcare provider. If the patient is willing to make a decision to work with the organ systems that remain intact, it is astonishing how the body can adapt. I am not trying to be foolish. There is a limit to what the body can do. Having surgical intervention with the removal of female reproductive tissue is attacking the nervous system of the body. Function will be permanently changed to some degree.

I just got off the phone with a very educated female from the East Coast asking how I could support her body with her ovaries removed. That is a huge dilemma. The body is designed to be self healing and can adapt to many situations. She may be required to take some type of ancillary supportive supplement for the duration of her life. However, if she modifies her habits, feeds the body so that it can detoxify itself and restores nervous system function through spinal corrective care, the body will adjust to the change and continue functioning. The real key is in creating the environment for optimal health. She cannot continue with the same self-destructive habits she had prior to the surgery or she will not see restoration.

I have practiced since the late 1970s, so you can say I have been back and forth down the "yellow brick road" of life a few times. I was trained to think of healing from the "inside out" versus from the "outside in." And, by the way, I have always been a natural doctor, long before it was popular. I was not trained with a western medical mind set of symptomatic stimulation or the suppression of bodily function. If you follow some basic natural principles of feeding the body right and stop dumping artificial foods into it, and restore the nervous system, the body will do everything it can to detoxify and heal itself. Our bodies are self-healing structures.

I would like to start this adventure by inviting you to participate with me on a journey as if you were one of my patients. Not all accept care because it requires change. Many have been invited; some have walked the road for a while and have gone back to their prior patterns. Others have stood fast, making an educated decision to be the captain of their own ship.

I am really fortunate because I have treated patients for a long time. The significance of that to you is that I have a pool of women who have implemented what I have written, and they don't or did not have hot flashes, tender breasts with menses, cysts on their ovaries, breasts removed and other common intervention. I have even treated patients who were diagnosed with cancer thirty years ago who chose to follow some logical suggestions and they are alive and well and approaching ninety years of age. I know natural care works.

I would like to help you navigate through this very exciting time in your life. You do not have to have fear of hearing the "C" word with a tear in your eye. I am going to teach you the basics; it is not complicated or mysterious. I will give you a logical approach to engage in your daily routine. Think of this book as your map to allow you to celebrate with your inner circle of friends, family, and children, grand and great grand-children. You are going to a new land and I am excited to have you on the trip. Get ready…because here we go.

Be Blessed

Dr. Bob DeMaria
America's Drugless Doctor

Introduction

MY ASPIRATION in writing this book is to reveal to you a potentially new set of thoughts and ideas, especially if this is your first time discovering the other side of medicine and/or a renewal of passion for natural health remedies. The reason I say "potentially new" is that you may have heard and read about drugless care but never really knew how to pursue it, and this is the first time you have reached out for something totally untested by your mind set.

I will look at your current body signals through your eyes—the patient. I have repeatedly witnessed that healthcare providers get so focused on what they do that they forget the patient is a person just like themselves. As you read the text with insight into the area of human female hormone physiology, I want you to know that I am listening and talking to you from these pages as if you were in the room with me. I feel your emotion of "Please listen to me." I know there is a natural answer. My main purpose in writing this book is to give you a breath of fresh air and HOPE. There are simple answers to your tough questions; I have been answering them in my natural practice for over thirty years.

What I want to share with you is very important for your long-term health. What I will be discussing is counter-culture. The good news is, there is a natural answer to your current situation. The thoughts and ideas that I would like to share are based on my tenured, clinically-based evidence and experience.

Honestly, today there are so many concepts and ideas used to treat people from the pharmaceutical and natural health fields it can be like going through a maze. I believe from what I see, hear and read that some of it can be an educated guessing game. Unfortunately, the lives of people are at stake.

I will keep the explanations as basic as I can. The biggest concept I can share with you is the fact that healing comes from within, no matter who you are. Long-term, optimal health will never come from a modality or treatment from the outside in.

When an idea is conceived it is called a thought; when a thought is conceived it is called a concept. We can only understand life to the degree that our concepts are correct. If an idea is wrong, the concept is wrong, and consequently, the understanding will be inaccurate and incomplete. You will suffer the consequences of the wrong concept in the health arena if it opposes natural principles. You won't respond long term regardless of your economic and social achievements. I have known billionaires who have died because they followed an incorrect treatment protocol.

The real reason why so many never achieve optimal health, regardless of the amount of technology, surgery and medication they undergo, is that they were lead to believe the wrong idea.

You are able to understand properly if your concepts are in alignment with your ideas, and your ideas are based upon truth. I am not sure if you have been told the truth when it relates to hormones in the female body. A number of the prescription treatment procedures that have been prescribed for hormone replacement are also on a list of carcinogens that cause cancer. Are you aware of that? It is listed on the American Cancer Society's Web site for the whole world to see. www.cancer. org/docroot/IED/content/PED_1_3x_Known_and_Probable_Carc inogens.asp?sitearea=PED. I think you will find it fascinating.

The chemicals listed are actually quite common. I suggest you may want to study the list. You may be exposed to some of these carcinogens, and you really need to avoid them. The most frightening to me is the synthetic hormone used to treat menopause. It does not make sense to me that a person would take a product known to cause CANCER.

Today the public is doing what they can to say "NO" to prescription medication. Whoever would have thought that there would be a proactive community looking for answers to their own health questions that did not include a prescription? We live in a very inquisitive time. A possible challenge is: Who do you believe? I always personally write to submit the true facts on natural healthcare.

So, let's talk a bit about the reality of what is going on out there in the real world. You see, everyday, I consult with patients who have been on the medical merry-go-round. They have frequently been coerced into radiation and chemotherapy when diagnosed with cancer. "This is the way we have always done it." This was what one physician recently told a new patient before she came into my office.

I also have had the pleasure of treating medical healthcare providers and physicians. Do you know what? They have the same issues as you do. There is no difference. The degree behind your name does not stop positive or negative physiology. In fact, I have often seen knowledge postpone necessary natural treatment. Healing always has to come from the "inside out;" not "outside in." This is a natural principle.

I have consulted with patients whose cancer has been placed at a level of ZERO, on a scale of one to four, and yet they were told they needed to put radiation and chemicals in their bodies. Rarely does it come up in my consultations with patients that their physicians ever discussed WHY they had the cancer and WHAT they could do?

Not too long ago, if a physician said anything against hormone replacement therapy, he/she was ostracized and thrown out of the hospital and out of the inner circle. Today, the "hip" physicians are suggesting herbs and creams, and unfortunately antidepressants. Ever since the government released the statistics on hormone replacement therapy and some of the side effects, women have been asking more questions.

The pharmaceutical companies and their representatives are ruthless in their desire to force information on the physicians while they are actively seeing patients. Do you ever wonder who gives the physician their information once they graduate? Do you know who pays for their Continuing Education Credit events? I have been to many medical events where there are HUGE numbers of physicians in attendance and guess whose banners are flying in the hallway? Yes, you guessed it…the pharmaceutical industry trying to woo the allopathic healthcare providers into using their products. It is not uncommon for one cholesterol lowering prescription medication to generate over TEN BILLION dollars in ONE YEAR.

OK, so what are we going to talk about in this book? I AM NOT GOING TO TALK ABOUT THE BENEFITS OF SOY AND BIO-IDENTICAL HORMONES. You won't need to find a compounding pharmacist who formulates designer hormones for you; the best pharmacist is living inside of you. Has anyone ever told you how to wake up the pharmacist in yourself?

I have charted a course with ideas and protocols that may not be a current standard, but nonetheless, has been proven by a positive track record over time by Natural Doctors. Thirty years ago everyone was told to use the low fat, trans fat diet, only to find out they were wrong. Remember this, and this is a very significant point: YOU CANNOT FOOL MOTHER NATURE!! The earlier navigators were in un-traveled waters more often than familiar territory, and lived to tell about it. Imagine listening to some of their wild adventures. Well, what I will discuss is not wild, but it is delightful to read the testimonies my patients have penned for you to read while they have been on the journey with me. We will be focusing on the following subjects:

NATURAL POINTS TO OPTIMAL FEMALE HEALTH

- Keep the **lymphatic** system moving.
- Clean the machine for optimal **liver** function.
- Stoke the **thyroid** to keep the fire going.
- Support the **adrenal glands** — your back up hormone system.
- Strengthen the **frame** and **structure**.
- Maintain the **communication** between the brain and tissue cells.

JUST TELL ME WHAT TO DO!

- What do I **eat?**
- How do I **exercise?**
- What **tests** should I have completed?
- How do I **change?**
- What **supplements** do I need?
- How do I get off my **medication?**

YOU ARE WHAT YOU EAT

- **Food Transition Guide**; steps to change
- **All about FAT**; you need the right fat
- **Sweet Alternatives**

I would encourage you to be open minded; some of the information I am going to suggest may be just the opposite of what you read in the magazines and popular newsletters from which you normally get your data. I am going to focus on what you need to do if you want to have optimal health.

I will be explaining the function of certian endocrine glands; such as the adrenal glands which are located on top of your kidneys, the thyroid gland found in the middle of your throat area, and organs like the liver which is a HUGE player in the whole process. From researching journal articles and listening to my patients, I have learned that there are patterns associated with certain conditions. If you can discover your pattern and change it, then you should be able to help prevent and correct a deficient or diseased state. The breast cancer pattern is a very important pattern to understand.

I would like you to know that habits formed when you were very young affect your menstrual and female health as you get older. Addictions to sugar, fries and chocolate at two years old can precipitate a lifetime of misery. I treat four and five generations of females. I see habits started with great grandbabies which are the same habits that are strangling the great grandmas. If you had menstrual issues your whole life, chances are you will have hormone challenges as you get older. That means, moms, your daughters may also have the same harmful body signals you have unless they heed your advice now. I know it is not always easy. Just because they are related does not mean they will listen. I have seen it in my own family. My mom has suffered with a lifetime of hot flashes, my sister had a hysterectomy in her forties, my mother-in-law had a mastectomy, and my niece suffers with menstrual challenges.

My wife had dysplasia (abnormal cells around her cervix) when she was thirty, that was the time we decided to make lifestyle changes in order to overcome this problem. She ate ice cream nearly every day as a teen, took the Pill, drank alcohol and ate fried foods like most others raised in her era. Her dilemma motivated us as a couple to do everything we could to help ourselves along with our patients. Eating organic whole food, weight training, aerobic activities and stretching became a part of our daily regime. As a result, her overall health has been awesome the last twenty years, without any significant female health problems.

I am not a Gynecologist, and I am not pretending to be one. However, I do understand physiology and know that if you can make lifestyle changes, you have the potential to get better. The resulting effects of stopping destructive habits normally promotes a healthy life. The quandary is connecting poor habits to poor health and providing a logical alternative and motivation to change based on results. Patients are tired of getting medical care that does not get to the cause of the problem. Often the side effects of medication appear to be more harmful than their benefits. I have successfully helped women who present themselves to my office with medically diagnosed conditions that have not responded to traditional treatment protocols. I treat them without using medications and/or special proprietary ingredients from some distant land.

It comes down to this basic plan: get the estrogen levels managed to normal in the ladies not yet into menopause, get the thyroid and ovaries fed the right nutrients and working as they are supposed to, have the colon evacuating freely, support the body after the onset of menopause by supporting adrenal function, and everything else will fall into place. We also need to correct spinal articulations and free up the communication between the brain cell and the cell tissues. I know it sounds easy, and guess what? It is! Once you understand what you need to do, you will smack the palm of your hand on your head and say, "I should have done this a long time ago."

I have spent a practice lifetime assessing saliva progesterone/estrogen testing, diet journals, thyroid panels, acoustic cardiogram graphs, symptom survey forms, spinal films, saliva zinc and pH screens, mineral tissue hair analysis, and countless hours in consultation with females of all ages and all levels of relationships, i.e., single, never married, divorced once, twice and many times, widows, pre-teens, teens, twenties to nineties. I have seen and heard a lot.

I will do my very best to create a whole new world for you IN SIMPLE TO UNDERSTAND LANGUAGE. Please DO NOT CHANGE ANYTHING immediately. This means do not go off your medication, have surgery or add more vitamin supplements until you read this entire book.

Then, I would pray for wisdom and crystal clear thinking as to what you need to do for your own situation. Your current health is specific for you; not your neighbor, sister, mom or best friend. You have your own unique circumstance. Yes, there are patterns; just don't do anything until you have discovered your own pattern.

Be blessed! It will get better, I promise. I have seen it happen for over thirty years, naturally…without drugs or surgery.

Dr. Bob

PART I

TEN NATURAL POINTS TO OPTIMAL FEMALE HEALTH

1
Hormones:
The Basics

I am sure by now you have read many articles about female hormones and/or listened to many of your friends, all trying to tell you what to do. There are days you may have cried what appeared to be gallons of tears because you think you are the only one with your condition (hot flashes, heavy menses, PMS, post-menstrual headaches, tender breasts, fibroids, etc.). No one seems to understand. You are mad at yourself, your spouse, best friend, neighbors, sister, high school and college friends, even your own mother. Heaven forbid if your husband comes home another night with a twinkle in his eye.

Your libido, which was once on fire, is waning and if you have one more night with a hot flash, you are going to move to Alaska and wait till this desert heat is over. You are beside yourself. I know; I've been there. Not in my person, but with thousands of females who have been through what I just described. I have talked to women who are very frustrated and confused. They just want someone to tell them honestly what to do. I mention all this because as a healthcare provider and husband who has been around a long time, I've seen and heard a lot. I have had conversations with many females who are tired of being led down a road they have no control over.

Hormones are a part of the many communication systems that help your body navigate through life. Think of hormones as messengers. Hormones are a part of the endocrine system that manufactures these messengers. There are organs that have receptors that are impacted by this hormonal form of communication and information, such as the uterus. Hormones are actually very potent concentrations, and when they are in balance, work awesomely. When you are under stress, overworked and do not eat the right foods, a puzzle is created that even the most astute endocrinologist (a doctor who works with the endocrine or hormone system) has a challenge figuring out, and many times does not. The whole body is interdependent on itself, which is why it is very significant when someone wants to have any organ or gland removed, especially an endocrine gland.

The endocrine system regulates the body's major continuous and prolonged processes

- Reproduction
- Growth and development
- Cellular metabolism and energy
- Blood balance of nutrients, electrolytes and water
- Mobilization of body defenses against stressors (things that cause wear and tear on the body's physical and mental resources).

The endocrine system is made up of eight different glands located strategically throughout the body.

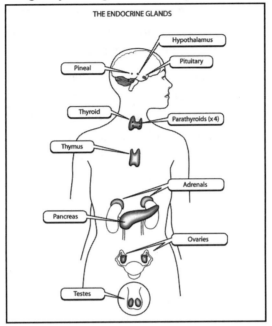

THE ENDOCRINE GLANDS

- Hypothalamus
- Pituitary
- Pineal
- Thyroid
- Parathyroids (x 4)
- Thymus
- Adrenals
- Pancreas
- Ovaries
- Testes

- The ovaries (in men, the testes) – source of progesterone and estrogen
- Adrenals (located on top of your kidneys) – makes sex hormones
- Pancreas islets (a part of your pancreas) – creates insulin and enzymes
- Thyroid (located in your throat) – source of thyroid hormone
- Parathyroid (a part of your thyroid mechanism) – assists in calcium function
- Pineal (in the brain) – has control of how light effects the body
- Pituitary – secretes many leading hormone activators
- Hypothalamus – the CEO of the body

Besides these major glands, the endocrine system includes pockets of hormone producing cells in tissues in the small intestines, heart, kidneys and stomach. The endocrine system develops and begins producing hormones by the end of the second trimester of fetal development.

It is safe to say that the endocrine system is probably the first system impacted by nutritional imbalances and deficiencies. Viable nutrients are needed to make and replace hormones, and the metabolic functions performed by hormones are nutrient based and mediated. That is why I see so many patients who wonder why they do not feel good, yet are eating convenience foods and are addicted to sweets, soda and novelty items. Your body takes what you give it and attempts to allow you to function optimally.

The hypothalamus is the commander and chief of your hormonal system. I like to think of it as the maestro. Have you ever been to a major orchestral performance? The maestro can take a collection of musicians who on their own sound great, but when you put them together with the right leadership, beautiful music results. It can create emotions that allow you to reflect on favorite times in your life. The hypothalamus connects the emotional and physical man. The hypothalamus controls autonomic reflexes such as the activity of the heart and smooth muscles. It houses the body's thermostat and biological clock, which maintains the body's rhythm of the twenty-four hour sleep/wake cycles.

The pineal gland also has a role in biological time keeping, being sensitive to retinal responses to light. The pineal gland is believed to coordinate fertility hormones and produces melatonin, the hormone known for its sleep triggering ability.

I suggest to my patients that wearing sunglasses can affect their health by altering the ability of light rays to reach the back of the eyes. When the adrenal gland is stressed, which is very common, the pupil or dark circle in your eye cannot stay small or constricted so light bothers your eyes. The adrenal gland indirectly has an impact on how the pupil operates. Wearing sunglasses inhibits the full spectrum of natural sunshine to enter the eye.

Do you sneeze when bright light hits your eyes? It may be another sign of adrenal strain. I know that the patients who enter my office with chronic health issues always have sunglasses in their purses, pockets or chicly placed on the top of their head. It is a consistent pattern and, by the way, the sunglass business is a multi-million dollar industry. We will talk more about that in Chapter Eight on the Adrenal Gland.

The hypothalamus also initiates the female cycle by producing gonadotropin-releasing hormone (GnRH), which signals the pituitary to secrete a follicle-stimulating hormone (FSH). FSH stimulates the ovaries to secrete estrogen, the sex hormone that stimulates development of breast, uterine and ovarian tissue (and the synthetic HRT forms are associated with excessive cell growth that leads to cancer).

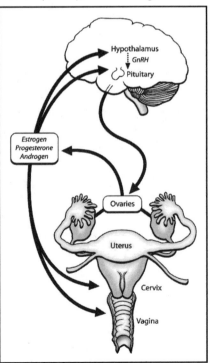

When estrogen reaches a certain level, it signals the hypothalamus to trigger the pituitary to secrete a lutenizing hormone (LH). Estrogen levels then fall, while the level of LH rises and peaks (around day 14 of the 28-day cycle), stimulating ovulation, the release of an egg from its ovarian follicle. I generally have seen very few females that have completed the saliva estrogen and progesterone assessments have a normal cycle. I have observed the peak of estrogen to be at all areas in the month. A critical issue with female hormonal health is the xenohormones; synthetic estrogen that is everywhere and literally is the key to the whole puzzle I will unravel for you.

After ovulation, the follicle (now called the corpus luteum) is filled with cholesterol, which is first converted to pregnenolone (a hormone precursor) and then to progesterone. The newly made progesterone is used, in part, for the building up of the uterine lining. If after about 13 to 15 days the egg is not fertilized, the uterine lining is sloughed off in menstruation when both estrogen and progesterone levels drop. Both estrogen and progesterone are necessary in the female cycle, and their BALANCE IS KEY FOR FULL HEALTH!!

Many women in our culture have an imbalance of these hormones, especially insufficient levels of progesterone to counter excessive estrogen—an imbalance that is further complicated by chronic stress, liver congestion and low levels of iodine resulting in a poorly functioning thyroid and ovaries.

Progesterone is a hormone important to a number of body functions. During times of stress or conditions of chronic adrenal hyper-stimulation, progesterone is capable of being converted into the stress hormone cortisol (natural cortisone, which helps take away pain and affects blood sugar stress). This explains why both men and women go to their healthcare provider tired and in pain, and find out their cholesterol is high. Your body is creating the cholesterol to help handle all the stress and inflammation in the body by being a precursor for your body's natural cortisone.

When one goes through chronic stress or severe, long-term stress, the hypothalamus will at first trigger an over production of the adrenal hormones; especially cortisol and DHEA (a hormone that helps make other hormones). This eventually leads to adrenal weakness, a state in which the exhausted adrenals cannot respond adequately. You're tired, bright light bothers your eyes, and you crave carbohydrates and salt (pickles, olives and chips). You may have also been told your blood pressure is low and, of course, your back goes out very easily. Does that sound like you?

The thyroid is also adversely affected by chronic stress. This gland's role includes regulating calcium metabolism and glycolysis (the breakdown of glucose for the body's energy and fuel). Under normal conditions, the fight or flight response from adrenal stimulation causes the thyroid to increase glucose breakdown. Glucose is the fuel to the system.

In conditions of chronic stress however, the thyroid is over stimulated and eventually becomes depleted. Cold hands and feet, HOT FLASHES, depression, constipation, thinning hair, morning headaches, thinning outside eyebrows, wide spaced teeth, and menstrual problems including scanty menses, sluggishness and high cholesterol are all body signals of a low thyroid. Thyroid function is also disrupted by excessive estrogen, but this can be prevented by adequate progesterone levels. Hyperthyroid (over active thyroid functioning) and especially hypothyroid (low functioning) have become more common. Adrenal and other hormonal gland dysfunction can cause some of the above symptoms and many more which will be discussed in more detail in the Adrenal Chapter.

One very damaging adrenal dysfunction is excessive cortisol production which causes, among other serious problems, increased calcium mobilization from the bones leading to osteoporosis, or loss of bone density. In a person with a healthy stress response, excessive levels of cortisol are automatically buffered. Constant stress destroys this feedback loop.

Hormonal imbalances compromise not only physical health but also psychological health, manifesting as problems ranging from depression to panic disorder. One way the body tries to compensate for imbalances created and exacerbated by the demands of stress is to over produce key hormones. Another way it tries to compensate is by converting sex hormones to stress hormones, thus further diminishing reproductive functions and the enjoyment of sexual health. This, by far, is one of the leading body signals that I see in my practice....the loss of sexual desire. If you do not have the desire or ability to engage in sexual intimacy, you probably have a severely drained system that needs to be recharged. This is very common in the dual income family, over-committed lives with our children, parents, co-workers and extracurricular events.

It will be very helpful to learn about these hormonal inter-dependencies because they allow you to see the bigger picture, and the problems commonly associated with menses or menopause are actually an indicator of a greater endocrine imbalance. For many women, the next step to understanding the bigger picture may be to look at their digestive health, including liver function and the foods that promote long-term cell efficiency.

THE PROBLEM WITH SYNTHETIC HORMONES

Hormones function much like a key mechanism with two ends on it. Let's call one end the R or receptor end. It fits exactly into a cell receptor and "unlocks" the metabolic door to start an action. The enzyme end, or E end, fits precisely with the cellular enzymes that transform the hormone into another hormone or into a metabolite for excretion.

When a synthetic hormone enters the cell receptor, its R end is similar to the real one, but not the exact fit. This jams the cell receptor or alters the action initiated. These are the reasons there are side effects from synthetic hormones. The synthetic hormone does not have the correct E end, so it cannot be properly cleared from the receptor, transformed into other hormones, or properly metabolized and excreted. This creates more bad effects. If you want to disrupt the delicately balanced endocrine symphony, giving synthetic hormones is an excellent way to do it.

This can even be more intense when the steroid system in the body is disrupted. The steroid system has its own interdependent melody that controls many functions in the body. The real issue occurs when synthetic steroid hormones are produced by the pharmaceutical companies. Today, in the natural care field, there are many who are suggesting the use of plant-based sources of "sterols" or natural plant-based ingredients to make female hormones to normalize function. Soy sourced bio-identical hormones are an example of these products. The pharmaceutical companies, on the other hand, have created a variety of items sourced from horse urine in attempting to normalize the imbalance in female hormonal health. The challenge with both attempts to help from this "outside in" approach is that they do not get to the cause of the problem. Granted there are individuals who do respond, and I would suggest they may want to stick with what they have going on, but I have consulted with many who, over time, begin having other side effects that generally involve menstrual flow, emotional swings, tender breasts and even upper respiratory irritation.

What synthetic hormones should you be aware of? There is a huge challenge with conventional hormone replacement therapy. No one in their right mind would think of taking a sophisticated jet aircraft in flight and entering alien commands into its computer control system. Yet conventional Hormone Replacement Therapy (HRT) does the equivalent of this when given to a woman. Alien (and therefore unpredictable and unknown) commands are entered into the endocrine or main "computer control system" of a patient through the drugs inaccurately called "hormones" used in HRT.

DESCRIPTION OF CONVENTIONAL HORMONE REPLACEMENT

Premarin (also called conjugated estrogens) is a word composed from Pregnant Mare's Urine. This horse estrogen is the most commonly prescribed estrogen in the world. It is also the form of estrogen most commonly used in research. This means that most of what we think we know about "estrogen replacement" in women is actually about horse estrogen "replacement" in humans. I have suggested as an experiment that you can take one of those tiny little yellow pills, add hot water to it and smell. Yes, you guessed right. You re-created horse urine.

In my practice we often use a quality source of Wheat Germ Oil® or Chlorophyll Complex®, which provides the proper nutrients; feeding the body what it needs to create the environment to produce estrogen naturally. I will be discussing in the Adrenal Chapter how your own body can make enough estrogen for your physical and emotional needs by supporting adrenal gland function. You see, when women are in their child-bearing years, they have an abundance of estrogen. As their nest empties, so does the natural time frame of abundantly flowing estrogen. However, in today's society and culture, women are now expected to be able to take care of grandchildren and great grandchildren. This creates an unnatural, stressful atmosphere and is a reason as to why we see health challenges in women who are raising their grandchildren. I see major burnout from over-expectation in many women. I am not suggesting that you go into seclusion. I am suggesting that you may want to evaluate the level of stress being place on your body. Many women today are also the major financial sources of income in matured families and relationships, and there are so many that are single due to divorce and death that have the additional burden of working forty, fifty and sixty hours per week; many times working three jobs. This creates an environment for physical melt down.

Estrogen is a steroid. Steroids are used to make natural cortisone. So, in essence, if you are stressed, eating sugar and nutritionally exhausted, I can almost guarantee you will have estrogen deficiencies.

The problem with Premarin includes the following possibilities. First it is for horses, not humans. The bad side effects include the following:

- Heavy menstrual bleeding, cramping
- Breast tenderness
- Fluid retention, edema, weight gain, increased fat storage
- Headache, migraine
- Depression, anxiety
- Glucose intolerance, Insulin resistance
- Estrogen dominance
- Stimulates growth of fibroids
- Worsens endometriosis
- Nausea, vomiting, cramping, bloating
- Leg cramps
- Eye problems
- High blood pressure
- Increases blood clotting tendency

- Venous thromboembolism, pulmonary embolism
- Increased risk of endometrial cancer and breast cancer
- Loss of scalp hair, growth of facial and body hair
- Gallbladder disease
- Pancreatitis

The composition of horse estrogen is vastly different from human estrogen.

HUMAN ESTROGEN	PREMARIN
Estriol 60-80%	Estrone 75-80%
Estrone 10-20%	Equilin 6-15%
Estradiol 10-20%	Estradiol & others 5-19%

The metabolic breakdown products of Premarin are biologically stronger and more active than the original horse estrogens. Various studies have shown that these breakdown products can produce DNA damage that is cancer-causing. So, for example, the incidence of breast cancer increases when women take Premarin. Premarin, like all conventional HRT, is prescribed in standard dosages and not tailored to individual requirements. This usually means women are often taking much more "estrogen" than they need. It takes about eight weeks to clear Premarin out of the body. In contrast, natural hormones are completely metabolized and cleared in 6-12 hours. Premarin can easily, and usually does, throw a woman into estrogen saturation or dominance. The word saturation is significant because there is just plain too much in the body. Outside sources of synthetic hormones create imbalances; it causes an excessive increase in Sex Hormone Binding Globulin (SHBG) which, in turn, blocks thyroid hormone function. You learn more about that in the

Thyroid Chapter. Estrogen and stress block thyroid function. This is all starting to sound like a very interesting puzzle, isn't it?

Progestins, another human knock off medication, is a chemical or drug imitation of progesterone, with its own set of negative side effects. PROVERA (medroxyprogesterone acetate) is the most common progestin. It is also used in PremPro, which is Premarin and Provera in combination. Most progestins are made by taking natural progesterone and altering the chemical structure so it can be patented. Another type of progestin is made by altering a synthetic form of testosterone.

Problems with progestins include suppressed production of natural progesterone in the body. It disrupts the steroid hormone pathways, which can cause both immediate and slow undermining of both adrenal and human hormone function. Since the steroid hormone pathway is fundamental to energy and vitality, this drug is usually a prescription for chronic fatigue commonly with patients that have inflamed tissues or the named condition: fibromyalgia. The myriad list of negative side effects includes:

- Depression
- Anxiety, nervousness
- Fatigue, leading to chronic fatigue over time
- Fluid retention and breast tenderness, weight gain
- Migraine
- Coronary artery spasm
- Angina, palpitations
- Menstrual irregularities, spotting
- Glucose intolerance; promotes insulin resistance
- General edema
- Nausea
- Insomnia, sleepiness

- Skin rashes, acne
- Hair loss on scalp, facial hair growth

There are potentially life-threatening adverse effects of progestins. Spasm of the blood vessels around the heart is the most significant. Some other life-threatening adverse effects are:

- Stroke
- Pulmonary embolism
- Implicated in causing breast cancer.

Ninety percent of men who have heart attacks have atherosclerosis or obstruction of coronary arteries, but only thirty percent of women do. The majority of women who have heart attacks do so because of coronary artery spasm. We use a product called Cataplex G® and Magnesium Lactate® along with strengthening the adrenal glands to protect against heart blood vessel spasm. In Chapter Fifteen on Tests, we also incorporate an assessment of heart sounds to determine what nutrients may be needed to promote natural function of the heart muscle.

Recently there has been information and statistics released about HRT and the link between discontinuing the use of synthetic hormones and the reduction of breast cancer. There is a lot of debate about the subject. As a result of my clinical-based experience, I am of the opinion that you cannot put synthetic hormones into a body, knowing the components do not match with the human counterpart and expect nothing to happen. I would not take any synthetic hormone regardless of how safe any drug manufacturer says it is. Historically, they have been wrong before, and they can be wrong again.

FACTORS THAT ALTER HORMONAL HEALTH

The physical condition of your mother and your birth order has an impact on your present hormonal health. Your birth order is important because if you are child two or three in the family order, the likelihood is that your mom had an overworked liver and fewer nutrients available to you. I really see this happen a lot in the patients who were the second child. If you were kept in the hospital or had to go back because of jaundice, it is probable you had a reaction with your mom's system. The liver is affected even before you arrive into the world. A congested liver from the beginning of life can be a challenge as you become a teen.

The amount of quality whole food oil your biological mother consumed also has an impact on your hormone health. That does not mean you cannot modify and alter your life now. I am making a statement of possibilities. I see patients of all ages that start life off with unusual circumstances. They may have had asthma or eczema from the very beginning of their lives. They then just seem to have a lifetime of hormonal health issues. I know that sexual hormones do not become evident until late adolescence, but your hormonal existence depends on many factors that are established very early in life. Even the fact if you were breast fed or not has an impact on your hormonal levels. You get more complete nutrients as a breast fed child.

A body signal for liver congestion I commonly see is freckles right below the eyes and on the nose when a child is anywhere from eight to ten-years-old. That is when the hormones start to kick in and the liver is working overtime to process them. Freckles, from my experience, are a sign of excess copper and not enough zinc. You should work on supporting liver function. Females who ate foods that were toxic to the liver when they were adolescent can continue their entire life with challenges since the liver has been under never-ending overload.

Freckles in adults are also a sign of high copper. Patients with high copper usually have high estrogen. High estrogen means thick and pasty bile. Thick and pasty bile may mean that you had your gallbladder out or someone wants to take it out. There are 500,000 removed every year as it is. Eating one-half of an apple daily will help. Apples have malic acid that will keep your bile moving.

Also, did you have mononucleosis when you were a teen? If yes, that is an important fact and raises the red flag of liver stress. The liver is important in processing all the used hormones, toxic foods, preservatives, medicines and other outside toxin in the body. Mono creates havoc on the liver. The liver is one of the main organs that has special cells that clean up toxic and foreign substances.

Would you believe that if you have had a lifetime of eating fruit after a meal that you could have liver stress? Yes, the fruit ferments on top of the food in your stomach. It is like having a constant drip of alcohol from the fermentation process going on. Your liver needs to process it. Has your life been a fog; poor memory? It is possible that your liver was over worked.

I have seen from my practice that when you feed the body correctly, your body will be able to make its hormones specifically for your needs. You cannot fool Mother Nature.

REVIEW OF SYMPTOMS AND CAUSES
OF HORMONAL PROBLEMS

The hormonal system is a communication system. There are eight organs associated with the hormonal or endocrine system.

- Stress can be the main cause of your hormonal issues by affecting the adrenal glands and the thyroid.

- Low blood pressure, wearing sun glasses, getting dizzy going from a sitting to a standing position and craving salt are signs of adrenal stress.

- Cold hands and feet, HOT FLASHES, constipation, thinning outside of the eyebrows, morning headaches may suggest a low thyroid.

- Cholesterol elevations can be directly linked to inflammation-causing foods like sugar and trans fat.

- Cholesterol will elevate when under chronic stress.
- Estrogen that is not balanced by progesterone can create hormonal imbalances and is the MOST COMMON CAUSE OF FEMALE HORMONAL issues prior to menopause.
- Xenohormones are common substances in our toxic environment that can create an estrogen dominance situation.
- A healthy liver is necessary to process toxic substances including medications, synthetic hormones and estrogen.
- What you eat has a bearing on your hormonal health.
- Processed foods, including trans fat or partially hydrogenated fat, congest the liver and lymphatic system.

NOTES_____

_____

_____

_____

_____

_____

_____

_____

_____

Patient Testimony:

"Before making Dr. DeMaria's recommended lifestyle changes, I had been dealing with some cysts accompanied by very heavy periods and clotting. Following his advice, I eliminated sugar – the desire for it gradually went away and I occasionally used soy. I gave up dairy for the most part and added flaxseed. Pretty much completely giving up the refined carbohydrates was the most difficult change.

Being a patient of Dr. Bob's has benefited me greatly over the many years I have been going to his office. Six years ago, I was told by my OBGYN that he would recommend laparoscopy to check one of my ovaries and possibly remove it. This was after MRIs, blood tests and ultrasounds proved negative. Dr. Bob gave me the confidence to say "no" to this unnecessary procedure. Changing my diet to eliminate sugar and dairy and to include flaxseed oil and food supplements everyday helped me greatly. Of course, the regular spinal adjustments were extremely important, as well, to keep my body running optimally. Today I still have two healthy, intact ovaries and have Dr. Bob to thank for helping me.

I feel healthier just coming to his office. The nutritional advice, adjustments, Standard Process supplements, encouragement from Dr. Bob and his staff all help. Additionally, my last menstrual period was 13 months ago. I feel great and am not bothered with any menopausal symptoms!"
Melanie McCrone

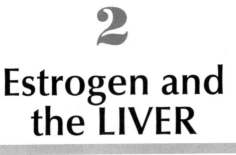

Estrogen and
the LIVER

A machine is dependent on all the parts working at one hundred percent. If one area is not up to par, the whole unit suffers. I was reading an article about the sport of rowing, or "crew." The athletes are in essence a group of very strong, high testosterone young men working as one contiguous unit. The difference between victory and second place is passion and attitude. If one team member loses focus for one stroke the whole team can be thrown off because that ONE paddle will cause the other members to lose synchronization and the other paddles will collide. The body is a little more forgiving. It will work hard and have another organ or system compensate — for a season.

My research indicates that there are two camps out there when it comes to the liver and how it works. Those that want you to buy their product to cleanse the liver/gallbladder mechanism and others who strongly have gone on record saying that cleansing the liver does not promote improved health. I have witnessed that individuals who avoid the toxins found in the food, water and environment have awesome results with their hormone issues versus those who continue on with unhealthy toxic patterns. They do not respond, even succumbing to surgical intervention.

It is not about taking another "all natural" remedy or a prescribed medication. It is about changing what you have been putting in your machine. You do not necessarily need something else, natural or pharmacological; you really need to stop challenging liver function with what you put into your body.

Here is the key. There are two main reasons for having hormonal issues before and after menopause. One is, before menopause you have too much estrogen and then afterwards you don't have enough once your menses stops. Your liver is the organ that processes the estrogen to be recycled or eliminated out of the system. If your liver is busy working on processing out the sugar, dairy and trans fat, how is it going to adequately be able to process the estrogen? Or if you are too stressed out, the liver is working to create the environment in the body to handle the stress versus fulfilling its job description. People often experience major sicknesses after stress. Superman Christopher Reeves' wife died shortly after he did; I am sure because of the enormous burden her system was under.

It is like this in any area of your life. If you spend most of your time on one area, another portion of your life will be limited. There is an axiom, "where your mind goes your energy flows." Your time could be consumed with painting, golfing, or crocheting, but your dishes and laundry are piled up. What do you do when you need to wear something or need something to serve a meal with? A thought pattern I need you to come to understand is your body needs to be in synchronization. You don't want your liver so busy and over working that it can not keep up. Your liver might be drowning in the waste that is gushing in to be cleaned up.

The liver has a plan to help clean up the burden of chemical toxins called the P-450 system. The challenge is that today in our society the liver has to process an abundance of chemicals and debris that have become a part of our "normal lives," not counting the extra burden you may give it because of choices that you make in "moderation." The phrase "eat in moderation" gets more people into an overload situation than can be imagined. Think about telling someone who is a heroine addict, "but only a little." Sugar (heroine) is one of those addictive items patients like to tell me they eat "only in moderation."

As you drive down the road smelling the fumes from vehicles, your liver needs to cleanse those fumes from your body or you would be a toxic dumping ground. Our bodies are relentlessly bombarded by what is invisible to the senses; chemicals that enter you through your skin, the water you drink and the air you breathe need to be transformed into non toxic substances. Daily patterns of living in our modern world result in a continuous flow of our own bodies having the impending ability to create toxic residue. These noxious substances can generate an environment for free radical formations. Think of free radicals as the rust you would see on a car or any metal object.

Free radicals are a part of the oxidation reaction that occurs when items deteriorate. Free radical production can create damage to fat and protein molecules in the body. This can also interfere with the production of the genetic make up of cells, creating the potential to have cancer growth in cells. This is a major reason why it is imperative that you keep exposure to toxins to a minimum.

Here is an experiment for you. Cut an apple in half with a sharp knife. Also, get a lemon. Cut the lemon, and squeeze some of the juice on one half of the apple. Wait about thirty minutes. Look at the flesh of the two apple halves. What did you notice? The side with the lemon juice should be whiter than the side without it. The brown color is oxidation. The lemon juice acts as an antioxidant preserving the apple. You will be slowing down the natural oxidation or rusting out of your own body when you eat blueberries and spinach, excellent sources of antioxidants.

This basic test will help to motivate you to avoid processed foods that would be similar to having your body oxidize, rust or decay, just like the apple.

The endocrine glands <u>secrete</u> hormones that are <u>excreted</u> by the liver or are chemically altered to make them water soluble so that the body may expel them effectively. The steroid hormones that are altered by the liver include estrogens, cortisol, aldosterone, thyroxin and others. The liver detoxifies or excretes these hormones into bile. Bile is also an antioxidant and a body degreaser. If the liver is not functioning properly, there may be an abundance of circulating hormones in the body at one time, leading to hormone over activity or toxicity. This excess of circulating hormones in the body will tax the endocrine system and cause other toxic reactions to occur such as too much circulating estrogen.

A part of this mechanism is the ability of the liver to properly metabolize protein; it is critical to your survival. The liver takes hurtful substances and makes them less noxious, with the help of protein, and then excretes them from the body. Think of the liver as the neutralizing agent by which toxins are neutralized. The liver also plays a central role in the synthesis of large amounts of cholesterol.

The liver is also in charge of the metabolism and storage of carbohydrates, as well as the assimilation and storage of the fat and water soluble vitamins. It is also critical for the storage of minerals. Now you can see why it is essential for the liver to remain in optimal working condition. Modern artificial toxins in the body can expose the liver to damage resulting in an inhibition of the cytochrome P-450 system and/or a decrease in liver metabolism ("sluggish" liver). Symptoms of such toxic damage include fatigue, hormone imbalance, increased fat stores, headaches, and blurred vision, etc., all associated with multiple health challenges.

The liver is responsible for more enzyme reactions than can be listed in this book. I want to make it clear that the liver is a very important part of the restoration of optimal female endocrine health. It is essential that you mentally absorb this information. In order to get to the root cause of pre-menopause estrogen saturation or dominance, your liver needs a source of whole food B Vitamins to properly process estrogen. This is very VITAL. What I have witnessed is that there is a widespread deficiency of B vitamins in our society. One of the factors that create a B vitamin deficiency is ingesting foods that are a poor source of B vitamins in the first place and then compounding the problem by eating products sourced from refined grains. The refined grains have had the very precious B vitamins extracted from them in the "processing" before being sent off to be used for animal feed instead of being used for human consumption. One other factor includes eating anti B vitamin foods, with sugar being the primary villain. Sugar depletes the body of B vitamins, and so does stress. Common symptoms of B vitamin deficiency syndrome include:

Apprehension	Noise sensitivity
Irritability	Acoustic hallucinations
Morbid fears	Tendency to cry without
Hypochondria	reason
Forgetfulness	Feeling something
Indigestion	dreadful will happen
Poor appetite	Weakness
Craving for sweets	Fatigue
Muscular soreness	Neuralgia
Depression	Neuritis

How many do you have? By far, the most common one I see nearly every day, and in all ages and genders, is crying without any reason. I also commonly see a fear of impending doom. If you suffer with six or more of these symptoms, my recommendation would be for you to first minimize the amount of refined grains you consume, reduce your sugar intake, and do what you can to minimize stress in your life.

One last point I would like to add. Do mosquitoes seem to think you are one big piece of cake or pie? Individuals who come into the office and say, "Dr. Bob, look at my arms and legs. The mosquitoes were out last night and I was the only one they wanted," are deficient in whole food B vitamins. There is something about having enough vitamin B1 or thiamine. Without it, it's as if you have a bull's eye on your skin. I encourage patients who are "bug bait" to take six to nine Cataplex B® a day, especially if they have other body signals of the B complex deficiency syndrome.

Some of the body signals that I see with individuals who have challenges with liver congestion and the P-450 dysfunction, including an inadequate amount of B-vitamins, are spider veins in the legs, varicose veins, hemorrhoids, bronzing on the body (especially the left cheek), gallbladder removal, a slightly swollen or boggy wrist and, of course, crying without reason. B vitamins are needed to breakdown or process estrogen.

I often see this typical history in women who have hormone issues: they are thirty-five to forty years old, have two children, and are slightly to moderately overweight with a fair complexion. They have uterine fibroids and there is a history of gallbladder removal. The gallbladder, by the way, is not the problem; the real concern is the the liver is so congested it's causing the bile to be thick and "sludgy."

By far, the most consistent pattern with liver congestion is gallbladder issues. When bile becomes thick and pasty, gall stones appear in the gallbladder. These obstructive lesions can impair the gallbladder's ability to secrete bile. They, literally, can plug the bile duct or tube from the liver into the intestines. Your body needs bile as a form of de-greaser soap. Fat needs to be metabolized.

When you have your gallbladder removed, you impair the body's ability to metabolize fat properly. Historically, a pattern I see in patients with gallbladder removal results in individuals who consequently breakdown with cardiovascular or heart disease and cancer. The removal of the gallbladder results in some very potential negative consequences. Gallbladder removal is a signal that your body is not functioning properly. It is imperative that you correct the foods you eat and the chemicals you put into your system.

If you have had your gallbladder removed, I would strongly suggest you eat at least one-half of an apple daily; preferably a sweet apple, versus a tart one. The information is from my study of Indian or Ayurverdic Medicine. It is better for your digestion. I use a product in my practice that is a source of bovine bile salts called Cholacol® (See Chapter Seventeen: Cleansing Protocols). I have my patients who have had their gallbladder removed take one Cholacol® a day with their lunch or evening meal and/or when fat is eaten. The next day I suggest two and on day three take a total of three. On day four go back to one. If you continue to take the same amount all the time your liver will become dependent on the product.

Your liver will continue to produce bile. The problem is that there is not a reservoir of bile in the gallbladder, so when you eat food that needs an extra "squirt" it is not there, so you will have incomplete fat metabolism. This results in an inadequate amount of oil that will be needed to be a base for hormones. Are you starting to see the picture? Don't give up because you have had an organ removed. Your goal is to eat the right foods as discussed in Chapter Fourteen, What to Eat.

ESTROGEN

I would like to discuss estrogen in more detail in this Chapter because I know that if you understand that estrogen needs to be processed properly, you can see the big picture of the whole puzzle.

Estrogen is one of the several female hormones that are a part of the normal female hormone cycle. Estrogen receptors are found through out the body. You may have heard of a term that I briefly mentioned already; estrogen dominance or saturation. That is when you have more than enough estrogen than your body needs in comparison to progesterone. Estrogen is normally balanced by progesterone. I discuss progesterone in the Chapter Eight: Supporting the Adrenal Glands.

Estrogen is the general term used for the several types of estrogen made by the ovaries, adrenal glands, liver, breasts and to a lesser degree the testicles. Estrogens are steroids. That means they have a particular chemical shape. Steroids, including estrogen and progesterone, can be made from cholesterol. Cholesterol is the building block for other steroid hormones including the pain relieving properties of cortisone. Cholesterol is improperly blamed for so many health issues, but in fact it is fulfilling its job description. The elevation of LDL cholesterol is because the body is in a state of inflammation, and the LDL cholesterol is putting out the fire.

There are three main Estrogens that I would like to discuss.

1. Estrone or E1. Five to ten percent of estrogen is made of this type. It is considered a very strong estrogen because of its ability to cause cell proliferation.

2. Estradiol or E2. Five to ten percent of estrogen is made of this type. It is considered the strongest estrogen because of its ability to cause cell proliferation.

3. Estriol or E3. Considered a weak estrogen because it does not cause cell proliferation. However estriol appears to balance the cell proliferation effects of estrone and estradiol, conferring protection against their cancer causing abilities.

KNOWN FUNCTIONS OF ESTROGEN

1. Confers female secondary sex characteristics
2. Promotes cell proliferation, especially of the uterine lining and breast tissue
3. Slows bone loss
4. Appears to stimulate and protect brain cells
5. Appears to raise HDL levels
6. Increases body fat
7. Creates progesterone receptors

SYMPTOMS OF ESTROGEN DEFICIENCY

1. Hot flashes
2. Night sweats
3. Insomnia
4. Mood swings
5. Mental fogginess, poor memory
6. Vaginal dryness, dry skin and eyes
7. Bladder infections
8. Incontinence, urethral irritations, urinary frequency
9. Headaches, migraines
10. Decreased sexual response

SYMPTOMS OF ESTROGEN EXCESS

1. Heavy bleeding

2. Clotting, cramping

3. Water retention, bloating

4. Breast tenderness, lumpiness, cystic breasts and enlarged breast

5. Weight gain

6. Post menstrual headaches, and migraines; one of the most common body signals I see in estrogen dominant females of undetermined origin

7. Depression, irritability, anxiety, anger

8. Decreased sexual response

9. When in excess, estrogen creates the environment for berry colored moles.

METABOLIC PROBLEMS THAT DEVELOP WITH ESTROGEN EXCESS

1. Loss of zinc, retention of copper (demonstrated on hair analysis and with the oral zinc sulfate test, available at www.DruglessDoctor.com)

2. Cold hands and feet, interferes with thyroid hormones

3. Impairs blood sugar control

4. Over time, increase the risk of auto-immune disorders

A couple of concluding thoughts: Estrogen only functions correctly when it is in the right proportion with progesterone, its primary partner and synergist. In a cycling woman, these proportions change; in menopausal women, the proportion of progesterone to estradiol falls ideally around 30:1.

Here is a topic that is not often discussed or understood. We have an over abundance of xenohormones which are a source of synthetic estrogens. The body is already dealing with a plethora of estrogen excess or estrogen saturation that is not being balanced with progesterone.

THE PROBLEM WITH XENOHORMONES

Xenohormones are man-made substances that are foreign to the body and have hormone-like properties. Most xenohormones have an estrogen-like effect and so are sometimes called xenoestrogens. This, in combination with a sluggish, physically congested liver, is one of the primary reasons why women in our society have so many menstrual and fibroid issues. Xenohormones can be absorbed by digestion, inhalation and direct skin contact.

COMMON SOURCES OF XENOHORMONES

- Synthetic estrogens and progestins, as are found in oral contraceptives and conventional hormone replacement therapies
- All American-grown, non-organic livestock, which are fed estrogenic drugs to fatten them
- Petrochemically-derived pesticides, herbicides and fungicides
- Solvents and adhesives (as in finger nail polish and polish remover, glue, cleaning supplies or industrial situation)
- Car exhaust
- Emulsifiers found is soaps and cosmetics
- Almost all plastics, given off especially when plastics are hot or are heated, (affecting meat and vegetables when wrapping with a hot wire at a meat department).
- Industrial wastes such as polychlorinated biphenyls (PCB's) and dioxins

DISORDERS RELATED TO XENOHORMONE EXPOSURE

- Increase in reproductive site cancers in women and men (breast, uterine, ovarian, prostate and testicular)
- Decreased fertility in both sexes
- Decreased sperm count in males, both human and animal
- Low testosterone levels and abnormally small penis size
- Increased incidence of undescended testicles
- Increased PMS challenges in women
- Estrogen dominance epidemic

STEPS TO AVOID XENOHORMONE EXPOSURE

- Avoid all synthetic and horse hormones (oral contraceptives and conventional HRT).
- Eat organic meat and dairy, and avoid the fat on non-organic meat and dairy, which is where the xenohormones concentrate.
- Decrease or stop all conventional pesticides, lawn and garden chemicals, etc. Don't contract with conventional lawn services that use sprays which are extremely toxic and full of xenohormones which add to our estrogen-saturated environment.
- Wear protective gloves and clothing when in contact with any glues, solvents, cleaning solutions that contain xenohormones.
- Avoid particle board, synthetic fiber carpets and fake woods as much as possible. The chemicals you smell are xenohormones. Think about that when you are around a camp fire or use a wood burner at home. I have patients that are sick all winter when they use a wood burning stove.

- You need to ventilate properly when in contact with any of these materials. Think ahead. For example, if you do install synthetic fiber carpets, do so when the windows can be opened—it takes months to air out the noxious chemicals.

JUST TELL ME WHAT TO DO

- The most important detail is not to complicate the treatment. The answer to your estrogen saturation is to simply change what you are putting in and on your body so your natural systems can do what they have been designed to do, function at the cellular level and heal itself.

- Do not have any major surgery completed unless all natural protocols are exhausted and given time to work. If what is occurring in your body is not impairing natural function, such as a fibroid creating bowel obstruction, be patient. Estrogen dominance takes time to normalize itself.

- Your focus should be on creating a menu that focuses on whole food versus processed items; see Chapter Twenty: The Page Fundamental Diet Plan.

- I would suggest that you minimize sugar, conventional processed dairy products and partially hydrogenated or trans fat that tend to congest the liver.

- Refer to Chapter Five on the Lymphatic System and start bouncing!

- Locate a quality source of whole food B vitamins. I use a product from Standard Process Labs called Cataplex B®. Look at the B Complex Deficiency chart on page 262. How many do you have?

- Review the labels of products that are around your house and what you put on your body. How many do you see that are toxic? Review the list of Carcinogens at the American Cancer Society's Web page www.cancer.org/docroot/IED/content/PED_1_3x_Kno wn_and_Probable_Carcinogens.asp?sitearea=PED.

- I would suggest you eat Dr. Bob's ABC's daily — Apples, Beets and Carrots.

- Eating cruciferous vegetables like broccoli, cauliflower, cabbage and Brussels sprouts will assist your body in eliminating estrogen.

- Drink water from a pure source.

- Eat organic food; minimize herbicides, pesticides and artificial chemicals. Review the American Cancer Society's list of carcinogens.

- I would avoid soy. Soy has estrogen properties and I have found through experience that it can create physiology issues in pre and post menopausal women.

NOTES_____

_____

_____

_____

_____

_____

_____

_____

_____

_____

FOR FURTHER INFORMATION, see *What Your Doctor May Not Tell You About Premenopause*, by John R. Lee M.D. and Jesse Hanley, M.D. Chapter 5. Also cited; Seminar information from Balancing Human Hormones By; Dr. Janet Lang 2002. Seminar information from The Doctor of the Future By; Dr. Stuart White 2007.

3
Progesterone

The hormone puzzle can be complicated. I was a guest at a friend's wedding some time ago, when I noticed a couple checking into the hotel where the reception was being held. The woman was walking with a cane. She appeared to be too young to have had a hip replacement, so I calculated in my mind that she must have been disabled because of Multiple Sclerosis. As fate would have it, I bumped into her and her husband at the reception. As we were having a conversation about the usual details of life, I just had to come out and ask her why she had the cane—it is the nature of my inquisitive spirit. She proceeded to tell me that she had been diagnosed with MS some time ago, and that she also had a history with leukemia and a few other conditions.

I asked her how long she had suffered, and she mentioned about fifteen years. The next question, which is significant, was: What was going on in her life when this all occurred? Was there a major stress incident? She confided in me that there had been, and proceeded to share with me that she had several miscarriages. She also had a hysterectomy since then with her ovaries removed. I bring all this up to you because there are some patterns that are significant that we need to discuss in this section.

One of the main roles of progesterone is to balance estrogen. It is also known that progesterone is produced by other tissues in the body including the brain and peripheral nerves, and as time goes on, I am sure there will be other areas discovered that produce it, as well. Over time, I would venture to say, that it will be discovered that steroidal hormones are produced in minute amounts by cell membranes. You may be thinking, why then do women have estrogen and progesterone deficiencies with menopause? My answer to you is the fact that these cell membranes produce the little extra that is required to help top off what the adrenal gland and ovaries are supposed to do, but when you have adrenal glands that are not up to par and ovaries that do not have enough iodine for function, then even the cell membranes can not make enough.

Going back to the wedding guest, here are some points I have noticed over time. Women that have a history of miscarriages tend to be low in progesterone with associated body signals of low blood pressure, bright light bothering their eyes and salt cravings—typical stressed adrenal challenges. Progesterone keeps the system intact so the body can carry the fetus full term. There are several possibilities someone may not be able to go full term. An auto-immune complex creating a poor environment is often a factor. When there is not enough progesterone, the body innately calculates that there is going to be a deficit. Rather than going full term, the fetus is released. I have found that women with a history of a miscarriage or two, or even three, also tend to be ones that develop multiple sclerosis, one of many auto-immune conditions. This woman fit this pattern. I want you to understand that this is not going to happen to everyone, but it is more common than you think. She also told me she had cold hands and feet. Those are common body signals for a low thyroid. The thyroid needs iodine and other nutrients to make thyroid hormone, as do the ovaries need iodine to assist in making progesterone. She had her ovaries out with her hysterectomy, probably because she did not have enough nutrients to have optimal ovary function. So the puzzle with progesterone is very big. It is essential to balance out the effects of estrogen, and to assist the body for proper function. Progesterone is a building block for other steroid hormones.

One last comment about the wedding guest. The leukemia, which was in remission, could also be a part of the adrenal gland scenario, because when the adrenals are not up to par, the lymphocytes are handcuffed and not able to function optimally. The adrenal glands are also a part of the system needed to create progesterone. What we are looking at is a mosaic of many tiny tiles that all need to fit together. This is often overlooked by the conventional medical thinking mindsets.

KNOWN FUNCTIONS OF PROGESTERONE:

- It is a natural muscle relaxant
- Balances the effects of estrogen
- Maintains the lining of the uterus, ripening it for possible pregnancy
- Stimulates new bone growth
- Helps burn fat for energy
- Is a natural antidepressant when balanced with estrogen
- May help against auto-immune disease
- Functions as a precursor for other steroid hormones
- Can increase libido
- Increases the sensitivity to estrogen receptors
- Is a natural diuretic
- Is preventive against breast, uterine and all forms of cancer
- Facilitates thyroid function
- In pregnancy, maintains the developing fetus

✝ Progesterone functions throughout the nervous system with functions that are not totally all known

You can see from the list that progesterone plays a critical role in so many functions in the body. Before I list the deficiency symptoms, I would like to share with you that I prefer to create the environment in my patients for their own pharmacist inside of them to create their progesterone versus applying a progesterone cream. I agree that most women need to have additional progesterone, and I am aware that there are many very fine healthcare providers that strongly suggest progesterone creams. However, by applying the creams and not altering your lifestyle, the patients will never get to the real cause of the problem. The food and toxins in our environment drain the body's ability to create the items it was designed to do.

I do not recommend progesterone creams unless someone is bleeding very severely and they need progesterone to balance the estrogen. Putting progesterone cream on your stomach, buttocks and breast may stop heavy flow, but will not get to the cause. I am not saying progesterone creams are wrong, but they do alter normal hormone physiology. What I normally see when I do progesterone and estrogen testing (and this correlates with body signals) is elevated estrogen compared to progesterone from the onset of the cycle. Progesterone normally does not reach the peak like it should at the mid to end of the cycle. Estrogen is normally high from the beginning of the cycle and may dip a bit in the middle. As a pattern, estrogen saturation or dominance creates the painful breasts, heavy flow and headache at the end of or beginning of the cycle.

As I have stated before, I have noticed that women who have a history of miscarriages tend to have low progesterone levels. Progesterone elevates during pregnancy because of many factors. If it is low, the body will release the fetus because all the factors are not just right for a full term.

Many of my patients tell me they always felt the best when they were pregnant. I believe their progesterone levels were at the high point of their lives and it just plain old made them feel good. The corpus leuteum and placenta take over and make progesterone while you are pregnant. They probably had an exhausted system normally, and their bodies were not capable of producing enough.

When your progesterone is low, your body will not have enough of a precursor to make the anti-pain and inflammation hormone, cortisone. When you are low in cortisone your hypothalamus, or CEO of the brain and body, will instruct more cholesterol to be made to create progesterone which is a precursor for cortisone.

Now, when you go for a blood serum assessment of cholesterol and it is above normal, it more than likely is because your body may need more progesterone to give you pain relief by fulfilling the need to make more cholesterol. Sugar creates a demand on the body to produce more natural cortisone. Are you beginning to see that it is more than not eating meat and cheese to keep cholesterol down? In many situations lowering your cholesterol is harmful to your overall long-term health journey. It may not appear that way, but if you have pain syndromes then you need cholesterol to make cortisone. I don't want you to go out and begin eating pizza to raise your cholesterol, but I do want you to know that it is the inflammation about which you should be concerned. This is a huge puzzle and you need to look at the consequences of all your choices and view this for the journey; not a short term dash.

SYMPTOMS OF PROGESTERONE DEFICIENCY

- Pre-menstrual syndrome
- Heavy bleeding
- Spotting

- Clotting, cramping
- Water retention, bloating
- Weight gain
- Headaches, migraines
- Depression
- Anxiety, irritability, nervousness
- Decreased sexual response
- Endometriosis and fibroids
- Breast tenderness, lumpiness, cystic breasts
- Infrequent menses

SYMPTOMS OF PROGESTERONE EXCESS

- Sleepiness
- Drowsiness
- Bloating, constipation
- Depression

I would like to point out that progesterone synergistically only functions correctly when it is in the right proportion with estrogen, its primary partner and synergist. In a cycling woman, these proportions change through out the cycle. In menopausal women, the proportion of progesterone to estrodiol falls ideally around 30:1. Remember estrogen is necessary to create progesterone receptors, and progesterone up-regulates estrogen receptors.

The levels of progesterone and estrogen are best tested by assessing the levels in saliva. These amounts are going to be the truest. Serum levels are also dependent on other factors and the hormones are bound with protein. I also correlate the amount of zinc and copper on hair tissue mineral analysis. I have found when copper is high, estrogen is high. When copper and estrogen are up, I generally correlate that with a female that is fair with freckles.

The freckles result because of the elevated copper. I see this occurring actually in about three consistent patterns. When a young male or female adolescent is transitioning from a child to an adult, the sexual hormones start to increase and the liver is not capable of processing them because of the long history of poor food choices such as a lifetime of pizza and fries. This pattern can be accelerated in individuals who are the second delivered in the birth order. The first baby creates an extra burden on the female, if the mother is not aware of her consumption of certain items like alcohol, fries, ice cream, partially hydrogenated oils or trans fats and is on prescription drugs. The liver will not be able to handle all the extra work and the estrogen and copper will go up. Finally, when a female has her second or third child she may get a bit overweight and stop exercising which creates stagnation in the liver once again.

As this process continues, these women often will have a history of gallbladder removal because when estrogen is high, the bile gets thick and sluggish. These patients have a history of digestive distress an hour or two after eating which is a common challenge because the gallbladder is not capable of releasing bile that is needed to break down fat.

I am sure you have seen by now that the puzzle of balancing human hormones is more than putting a patch on your body, or taking one pill and expecting everything to get better. The success of your long-term health rests on the fact that you will need to make some pretty dramatic changes if you are facing ablation, hysterectomy or gallbladder removal.

JUST TELL ME WHAT TO DO!!

- Have your blood pressure taken lying down, then standing; if it drops ten to fifteen points, you will want to go to the Adrenal Chapter Eight and support the Adrenal Gland so it can do its part to create progesterone.

- Take your armpit temperature first thing in the morning for ten minutes, three days in a row. If the reading is less than 98.7°F, I would suggest you find an experienced healthcare provider that knows how to support thyroid function, and make sure you have the TSH, T3 and T4 tests done. You may need extra iodine, which feeds the ovaries, assisting in the production of progesterone. See more about the Thyroid in Chapter Seven.

- Have you had a history of miscarriage? If yes, you may want to do a saliva test for progesterone and estrogen. If you find the progesterone is low, that does not mean you need progesterone cream. You want to make sure your adrenals are functioning, the thyroid is up to par and your liver is doing its job. Study the liver, thyroid, adrenal and cleansing in Chapters Six, Seven, Eight and Seventeen.

- I suggest whole supplementation for the ovary. First, always have appropriate tests done: saliva for progesterone/estrogen, a thyroid panel and hair analysis to assist your decision on which organ you need to support. Generally, I will recommend a few different whole food products. First, I generally suggest and find the need is for iodine. I use Prolamine Iodine® up to twelve milligrams a day from Standard Process Labs. The iodine will assist the ovaries to make progesterone. Also, I may use animal sourced proteins called Ovex® (which will increase progesterone and not estrogen) or Ovatrophin® depending on the body signals of the patient. If there are symptoms of estrogen dominance, like tender breasts and heavy flow, I use both items just mentioned any where from six to nine a day for several months. This helps support progesterone production. I have used Chasetree® a product from Standard Process Division called Medi Herb. Chasetree® is an herb that assists ovarian function.

✝ I do not recommend progesterone cream, unless the patient is to a point of losing her uterus. My experience suggests that when you use progesterone cream you are literally hampering your body's ability to make its own progesterone. The feedback mechanism used by the brain/tissue loop to assess the amount of progesterone is being altered, even if it is natural progesterone. I always like to get to the cause. I am not telling you to stop using the cream. I am suggesting you think about the big picture. Your thyroid, adrenals and liver may need to be supported. Using the cream may give you temporary relief but is it helping in the LONG TERM?

✝ I would strongly suggest you find a skilled, experienced spinal-adjusting, nutrition-focused chiropractor. They could be the answer to nearly all of your issues, as I will discuss in the Communication Subluxation Chapter Ten, because your ovaries may not be getting the messages the brain is sending to them. The ovaries have a nerve supply. The nervous system does control function. I will discuss elsewhere in the book that I have seen health improve by correcting the spinal area directly associated with innervating or connecting the brain instructions to the ovaries, resulting in improved hormonal function. Releasing the subluxation by spinal correction is like turning the breaker back on to your appliance in your house or apartment.

✝ Always think about the liver. The liver is critical for proper hormonal function. If the liver is not doing its job, then estrogen will be up and progesterone will be down. You do not want that since your body will have a hard enough time trying to balance all the man-made xenohormones, which create the estrogen dominance scenario. Eat Dr. Bob's ABC's every day: one-half of a sweet apple, about one-third of a cup to one-half of a cup of organic raw, grated or baked beets and several baby carrots.

NOTES_____

_____

_____

_____

_____

_____

_____

_____

_____

Patient Testimony:

"Before making Dr. DeMaria's recommended lifestyle changes, I had been dealing with emotions of all sorts during my monthly cycle. Since modifying my sugar consumption and eating healthier, I no longer struggle with these symptoms. I feel better all over. I feel like I can breath easier, and I also sleep better.

I appreciate Dr. Bob's willingness and his enthusiasm in everything that he does. He is full of Godly wisdom and I am blessed to have him as my doctor." **Jennifer Traxler**

4
Other Hormones
Affecting the Balance

There are several additional hormones that I would like to discuss that effect the balance of female hormones. Xenohormones, which were discussed in Chapter Two on Estrogen, are by far the most serious of all hormones, and even though they are man-made, they are a part of the whole imbalance.

The items I would like to discuss include DHEA, testosterone and the synthetic chemicals that have been developed to replace or support the chemical messengers you already have in the body, i.e., conventional hormone replacement therapy (HRT).

DHEA stands for dehydroepiandrosterone. Pronounced dee-hi-dro-epp-e-an-dro-stehr-own, DHEA is a steroid hormone that helps build structure and is classified as an anabolic hormone. It is an androgen steroid produced by the adrenal glands, the ovaries and testes. Men normally have a slightly higher amount than women.

DHEA plays a role in energy, handling stress, mood and immunity. It works inversely with cortisol; when one goes up the other goes down. It can be used to cushion the ill effects of excess cortisol. DHEA helps decrease insulin resistance.

SYMPTOMS OF DHEA DEFICIENCY

- Memory difficulties
- Lack of stamina

- Lowered mood, depression
- Decreased sex drive
- Fatigue and exhaustion
- Inability to handle stress
- Impaired immunity

SYMPTOMS OF EXCESS DHEA IN FEMALES

- Irritability, edginess when the dose is too high
- Acne, oily skin
- Increased facial and body hair
- Found in women with multiple cysts on the ovaries

I generally do not supplement with DHEA. I have found it is better to support the whole body and adrenal glands, and work on eliminating stress and toxins so the body can restore its own levels. When DHEA first became popular, I had several patients that required quite a bit of time to stabilize their hormones after saliva testing showed they were overdosing on DHEA supplements taken on the advice of other practitioners. You can create quite a disaster of your own hormones by trying to increase one area without taking into consideration all of the ramifications.

Testosterone, mostly thought of as a male hormone, is also present to some extent in the female body. Testosterone is a steroid androgen hormone produced in small quantities in the ovaries and adrenal glands. It is made from the precursor progesterone and DHEA in the steroid pathway. Testosterone is an anabolic hormone, which means it helps build body structure.

TESTOSTERONE IN FEMALES

- Maintains sex drive
- Promotes healthy muscle
- Strengthens bone
- Helps mood and well being
- Maintains stamina and overall energy

TESTOSTERONE DEFICIENCY BODY SIGNALS

- Poor muscle tone
- Low or absent libido
- Decreased stamina and energy
- Decreased armpit and body hair
- Weakened bones, osteoporosis

TESTOSTERONE EXCESS BODY SIGNALS

- Acne, oily skin
- Loss of head hair, male pattern baldness
- Excessive body hair
- Aggressive behavior and disposition
- Deep voice

Low testosterone can be balanced by focusing on taking stress off the adrenal function and making sure the liver is doing its job clearing synthetic hormones, which create a potential hormone imbalance.

NOTES_____

_____

_____

_____

_____

_____

_____

_____

_____

5

Let's Talk About the Lymphatic System

The lymphatic system is probably one of the most mysterious systems in the body. You really only hear about it with an exercising rebounder enthusiast that bounces daily to get the clear lymphatic fluid moving or, unfortunately, from the cancer patient that has been advised by their physician that the cancer has spread to the lymph nodes. The oncologist (cancer physician) usually would say something to the effect, "It appears that the chemotherapy and radiation only contained the cancer for a while." Heart-wrenching words to hear echo through the cortex of your brain.

I would like to introduce you to the mechanics of the lymphatic system. It is literally the sewer system in your body, and it would be in your best interest to take care of it like you would the down spouts on your home, the drain in your bath tub or shower and/or the road gutter in front of your house. The lymphatic system is a network of channels that are multi tasked in nature. It is one of the several lines of defense of your immune system as well as the freight train hauling around fuel in the form of food particles. It is like the "Patriot Missile" line of defense, the infantry and supply chain all in one package.

The lymphatic system carries proteins and fats for digestion and activates lymphocytes (a type of white blood cell warrior). The lymph nodes in a person's neck, including the tonsils, swell and get red when they are DOING THEIR JOB protecting you. Having one's tonsils removed is like disarming a warrior or cutting the wire to the "warning signal" on your dash board. When we are born, there should be little tags on all of our organs that say "DO NOT REMOVE!"

I know we have been told that organs that are commonly removed are not necessary for life. I believe as time goes on we will hear more and more about the negative effects of the surgical removal of lymph tissue. The tonsils are the storage house mechanism of sulfur in the body. Sulfur is needed to help maintain cartilage for your structural health. A great natural source of sulfur includes eggs, onion and garlic. If your lymph nodes are swollen and sore, limit dairy, exercise your muscles and drink more water. It is very important for you to come to the understanding that when these and other tissues in your body are performing their job description you DO NOT REMOVE THEM!!

Lymph health is promoted by drinking water, increasing activity and avoiding processed foods and dairy. If your lymph nodes become swollen and sore, usually it is because you are consuming something that is overworking the system. If you continue to do that long enough you will get some type of chronic condition, including CANCER. Your children are no different. If they continually have swollen glands, DON'T GIVE THEM ANOTHER ANTIBIOTIC. Stop feeding them SUGAR and DAIRY. I also encourage lymphatic drainage massage by an experienced massage therapist. It will assist your body's line of defense and create open drainage for toxins that have accumulated in your tissues.

There is a term I think you will find significant and should be a part of your wellness vocabulary. The word "stagnant" is an expression that you would like to avoid throughout your organ systems, but most importantly in the lymphatic network. When the lymphatic system is stagnant, you are not going to be working at one hundred percent. You really want to keep all the fluids in your body moving at a nice rate, with no congestion or bottle necks. Some of the primary reasons I see a sluggish or stagnant lymphatic system is over-indulging on dairy sourced products, insufficient water in the diet and lack of muscle moving exercises. You want motion. Motion is life. It is easier to move clear lymphatic fluid versus the sludge created with inadequate water consumption replaced by a diet containing soda (diet soda included), power drinks (loaded with chemicals) or alcohol and coffee.

The cells in your body are analogous to machines, all working together for the good of the whole. When a machine is operating, there is generally some scrap or waste from the manufacturing operation. The maintenance crew commonly comes by and picks it up to go to the recycle bin. There is waste or a by product of production. Your cells have waste, and a part of the waste disposal system is your lymphatic channels in and around your arms, legs, neck, trunk and abdomen. The wastes are eventually going to be processed by the liver, kidneys and colon for recycling or elimination. Your colon, by the way, has one of the largest concentrations of lymphatic tissue.

The lymphatic system is also the organization that creates the warriors or lymphocytes that seek and destroy foreign invaders or cells that have become abnormal for whatever reason. The lymphatic system is similar to the maintenance crew; sweeping, cleaning and disposing. It is like the street crew in your neighborhood that cleans the streets and trash, often when you are sleeping in your cozy bed, but the lymphatic system is only capable of handling so much at a time. If the channels used to carry away the debris are so congested from over production or faulty disposal, it can get backed up.

I see it where I live when there is an abnormally large amount of rain. The gutters and down spouts on a house can only handle so much rainfall in a limited time period. If you failed to clean the gutter out, or there are leaves and sludge that have accumulated, you can be in trouble. There can be water damage inside the house and an overflow in the basement. I know from experience that this does happen, and generally read about it in the newspaper when the citizens in our community are upset with the city street and sewer department for not doing their jobs.

Another situation would be if you have two pumps working very diligently during a downpour, and you are feeling really good about the situation and all of a sudden you hear a crack of lightning and the power goes off. If you did not plan ahead with a battery backup pump or gas powered generator you can have a HUGE mess in the basement.

The outcomes of the scenarios that I have just described can be controlled. Now, you cannot control the amount of rain, but you have control over the way the water is disposed. Your body is no different. You cannot necessarily control everything that is thrown at your body, but you do have charge over what you do with it. And honestly, you really do have control of the majority of what goes in, even the level of toxins. Let me explain.

First, you want to make sure you are drinking enough water everyday. How much is enough? Well, the least amount you should drink is a quart. A general rule of thumb is to drink one ounce of water for every pound of body weight. I personally would not drink over one-hundred ounces a day, especially if you start noticing leg cramps at night or when you are walking. You would be getting rid of too many minerals. As I mentioned before, and this is important: avoid using soda, fruit drinks, energy drinks and coffee as your main beverage. Eat veggies and fruits as they have high water content. Avoid pastries and goodies that draw water out of the system to be processed.

Your colon is a dehydrator. If you continue to eat certain foods, especially wheat based items, you are creating coverings on intestinal walls that are thick and pasty. Your body needs water to cleanse the system. The next time you are hungry, instead of grabbing a "little" piece of cracker, cookie etc., drink a glass of water or have a piece of cucumber, a small tomato or piece of celery. You are putting fluid in which is positively proactive for your long-term health, instead of creating a negative state.

You want to make sure you are exercising. A re-bounder (small mini-trampoline) works by creating a vacuum in the lymphatic channels. This creates movement of fluid. Motion is Life. Your lymphatic system does not have the privilege of having its own pump like the cardiovascular system does. Any type of exercise is better than being a couch potato — walking, riding a bike, fast stepping or dancing.

I have several massage therapists that assist me in my clinical setting. They complete therapeutic massage treatments. One of the recommended techniques that they have all specialized in is lymphatic drainage massage. I have had patients who had swelling in their bodies diminish after having their lymphatic system properly stimulated and drained. I recently presented a workshop to my patients on skin health. I made a comment that the average Western female absorbs, either through friction or natural lip licking, up to four or seven pounds of lipstick over their lifetime. The massage therapist in attendance said she thought about what I had said and continued to tell me that she has noticed that when a female patient comes in for lymphatic massage and has lip stick on, that normally when the session is complete the lipstick or lip gloss is absorbed. She theorized that she was stimulating the flow of lymph fluid in the body. I thought that was a very interesting observation. I have not read or heard that before. I think that most people who have dry lips don't realize that it is an internal problem. Dry lips are a possible signal that you may need to increase your water consumption. Most would not think of the lips as a tissue directly linked to the lymph channels. If you are a massage therapist and you do lymphatic drainage, observe that phenomenon and let me know if you see the same thing.

The lymphatic system is not the bad guy. It is critical for your optimal health. Your objective is to keep the lymph channels flowing flawlessly. I have observed, in case histories, that patients generally have a long history of poor diet choices. I have seen this thousands of times as I review the food journals of my patients. Consumption choices focused on foods that do not promote regular, timely, no assistance needed bowel movements (that means without a laxative, natural herb, etc.), mostly concentrated on refined grains and starches. They have toxic looking skin, which is pale, not pink and vibrant, with many red and brown marks, varicose and spider veins. Little or no exercise is common on the intake history. All of these result in a stagnant system trying to get rid of the excess scrap from production.

The body is overwhelmed; it does not know what to do with all the excess. The environment in the body is at a point of what a toxic pond or river would look like. Cells begin to break down, and there is cell membrane destruction, oxidation, which is like massive rusting away. You can slow and stop the oxidation process, which is like the deterioration progression of steel, by increasing your consumption of veggies during the day. Veggies and fruits are like Rustoleum® and combine with the "free radicals" theorized to be in the process.

The tremendous magnitude of oxidation creates the potential for free radical or abnormal cell activity. The hormonal levels are everything but normal. You do not feel good for some time and finally start to have symptoms. A lump might appear on your breast, your menses is heavy, and you feel nauseated. Finally, you visit the doctor and many tests are completed on you. Then the time of the consultation — and you are told you have CANCER.

You make an appointment for further testing with a cancer specialist who decides to do a biopsy. You wait with baited breath for the results. You are receiving well wishes from friends and family, e-mails from people with advice on what to do, and finally you are told the cancer has spread to your lymphatic system. They want to take the nodes out. So now what do you do?

Here is my advice to patients. This is what I say every time, as diplomatically as possible. If you don't change what you are doing, you will DIE!! That usually gets their attention and a tear. I am not trying to be abrasive. You are in a battle. You are the "commander and chief" of your army. What you decide to do affects the VICTORY. You need to take responsibility to fight your own war. What you have done to this point in your life is the reason you are in the situation you are dealing with now.

The big question is: What do you do about the chemotherapy and radiation treatment? My suggestion is, to ask yourself how bad are the symptoms you are experiencing and what stage is the cancer? Sometimes, if the cancer is advanced, you may need the extra help to get it under control while you are making lifestyle changes. I would locate the book, *The Answer to Cancer* by Dr. Hari Sharma. He details what your steps should be if you are going to have chemotherapy. If your cancer is not advanced, then you have a fighting chance to win the war. I see it all the time in my natural drugless practice. I have had new patients present themselves at my office with tears in their eyes, make the decision to CHANGE, and they LIVE. I do not heal them. Their own body does the healing. I coach them. Unfortunately, many come in after the conventional methods have been exhausted and there is nothing else they can do; hardly a time to start thinking about making lifestyle changes.

Let me be candidly honest with you, and this is not meant to be unkind to the established way things are done in our society; but chemotherapy and radiation are not the ONLY answer. Those modalities and forms of treatment do not get to the cause of the problem. They are treating the symptoms. CLEAN MACHINES WORK BETTER. You need to clean the machine. Synthetic HRT treatment for female hormonal issues was standard by the medical community and women were dying because of synthetically-sourced, horse urine-based medication. It was extremely significant that the results of a government study were released in 2003, or the drugging of women would have continued. But now, it was recently reported that HRT is safe and effective for select age groups and stages of hormonal change. Do you understand how IMPORTANT this is? The battle you are in is for your own LIFE.

JUST TELL ME WHAT TO DO!!

- Focus on whole foods that promote bowel movements. Mixed greens and mostly raw (lunch) and steamed (dinner) vegetables should be a regular part of your diet. If you can't handle the taste or texture of raw which is common in patients who are really very acidic in their saliva pH, (See pH in the Testing Chapter Sixteen) eat steamed vegetables until your body can handle raw ones.

- Drink water as your beverage of choice. Avoid processed, pasteurized, homogenized, physically altered dairy, which tends to plug the lymphatic channels. Avoid eating cheese on a regular basis. According to the senior massage therapist on staff at my office, it creates a layer of palpable fat under the skin. She also noted that her clients who are regular cheese consumers, have a peculiar odor to their skin, especially their feet.

- Exercise your muscles regularly. That means some body part daily. Bounce on a large 55cm exercise ball or mini-trampoline.

- Stretch your muscles with flexibility exercises using an elastic band.

- Tonsils removed? Eat eggs, onion and garlic which will provide sulfur. The tonsils are your body's sulfur reservoir. An organic egg a day is safe and good for you. Eat the yolk. You do not need to have toast. Poached, hard boiled or scrambled with olive oil. Put some spinach in the egg, throw in some onions, and what the heck — add a dash of garlic!

- I would eat Dr. Bob's ABC's every day. One-half of a sweet apple, several pieces of baked or grated raw beets and several small organic baby carrots or a large peeled one that has been cut up.

- Start your day with a wedge of one fourth of an organic lemon with pure warm or hot water. This is good for the liver and digestion. I personally would eliminate the consumption of soda and alcohol, and limit coffee consumption. Soda has man made chemicals that stress the liver and kidneys. Alcohol, including wine (a media beverage for heart health), even in moderation is still processed, often with sulfates. I know that the literature says it will help your heart, however, eliminating the deserts and the wine with a meal will promote more life than drinking a glass of wine. Just a suggestion. Patients who have the discipline to curtail alcohol will lose weight, lower their cholesterol and get over depression quicker than the ones who hold on to the "moderation" theory. I see it in my practice routinely.

- Seek out a skilled massage therapist who is trained in lymphatic massage.

NOTES_____

_____

_____

_____

_____

_____

_____

_____

Patient Testimony:

"When I first came to see Dr. Bob, I had been dealing with a heavier flow, cramps, heart palpitations, psoriasis, mid and lower back pain and depression. I had been taking antidepressants, anthistamines, nasal drops and using psoriasis creams. Losing my mother was very tough on me physically and mentally, so my daughter suggested that I try Dr. Bob and see what it was like. I am still working on taking sugar out of my diet, and I take 1½ tablespoons of flaxseed oil daily. The most difficult challenge has been to really look at labels and know what to look for, especially hidden sugars.

After receiving my first adjustment and having my "switches turned on," I felt like it woke me up to a new happier person. I have never looked back. The knowledge and the adjustments have definitely helped me."

S. Dietz

6

Importance of Optimal Liver Function

Improving health at any level whether it be an adolescent with an acne issue, a teen with chronic headaches, a depressed twenty-year-old, a gallbladder that is congested and needing attention, along with a heavy menstrual flow, tender breasts or chronic pain syndromes—and I could go on—it all boils down to this question. Is your machine clean? So, Dr. Bob, what do you mean by clean machines?

I discussed how significant the lymphatic system is to the body. It is the sewer system, and basically, the clean-up crew. One major reason that females have health issues with their hormone function is because the body is not capable, at our current level of toxic overload, to handle what it is being exposed to.

Estrogen, as you are now aware, is one of the key hormones necessary for the female menstrual cycle. Estrogen elevates. When its purpose is complete in the menstrual cycle, it then gradually declines in strength and amount, with progesterone stepping it up and taking the dominant position. The lining of the uterus is sloughed off and the whole process starts over; easy, right? Not hardly. Estrogen dominance is the key reason most females suffer with so many challenges up to cessation of menses, and not enough estrogen being produced by the support organs is the reason they have severe menopausal problem after menses has subsided.

The liver's purpose as an organ is multifaceted, with hundreds of known functions for the body. It is likely that we will never know everything it does. Our understanding of the liver increases as technology uncovers more possibilities. Western mindsets think differently than other cultures when it comes to whole body function. Healing comes from the inside out, versus the premise that disease is something that comes from the outside in. Your body does have to deal with all the outside toxins, but most of them can be handled if the inside tissue is up to par and not over-stressed by toxic choices.

In other parts of the world, the liver is metaphorically exchanged for the heart that we so revere in our western culture. Can you imagine receiving a Valentine's Day card with a liver on the front instead of a heart? The liver is associated with anger in Chinese medicine, according to Jack Tips, PhD, author of *Your Liver Your Lifeline*. I often wonder if this is why we have road rage. People are racing and eating some of their main meals in the car. When I am driving around in town and on the highway, I see burgers in one hand, a soda in the other, along with a "Blue Tooth" ear piece, and down the road, a handful of fries being scarfed down in between sips of a diet beverage. As a society, we are literally trashing our livers with bad eating habits and choices resulting in a plethora of physical and emotional consequences.

The word melancholy can be traced to the term "bad blood." People who have congested, overworked livers tend to be more easily angered; a common body signal that I notice in many new patients. When I complete an assessment with various diagnostic modalities, liver congestion is generally evident with individuals who have shorter tempers. If you have a history of gallbladder surgery, which, by the way, there are over 500,000 of them a year, it is a sign to me that your liver is not up to par. Taking synthetic, high potency B vitamins can compound the problem and make the situation worse. I have seen fibromyalgia clear up in females when they get off their high potency, synthetic B's.

I was at an event recently when a professional colleague approached me with questions about his wife in her middle 50s. He was beside himself; he was doing everything he could to help a chronic health situation which included female body signals (tender breasts, heavy menstrual flow, PMS, post menstrual headache, spider veins on her legs and thighs), plus constant mid back pain. His wife then had some discussions with me and decided to come to my office for an assessment. During our conversation, she let it be known that she LOVED SUGAR. Sugar is the stealth player in our society that depletes the body of much-needed nutrients for optimal body function. I talked to her just as I am talking to you right now.

I told her, "Sue, you really need to clean up your liver, eat more veggies and drink more water." Her response, "Dr. Bob, I do all that, I have taken tons of supplements and did bio-identical hormone replacement, all without any change. So what else can I do?" It is not about what else to take, but what you should avoid. Anytime you consume a food that has been processed, your body actively needs to do something with it. Your body can only work with what you put in it. When you eat food, it does more than provide calories. Food creates the building blocks for life. Sue, like so many women, will not progress past where she is unless she avoids items that stress the detoxification system. I instruct my patients to minimize products that are highly processed or have a potential to be toxic. This includes over-the-counter and prescription medications along with synthetic vitamins which are stressful to the system.

In the owners manual for a vehicle, it is suggested that you replace your oil, gas and air filters on a more frequent schedule when you are in dusty conditions that create stress on the designed cleaning mechanism. The oil in those environments actually gets dirty and "gunky" quicker. There are several protocols that I recommend for liver/gallbladder cleansing. These are sensibly affordable procedures with a special bonus of being non-invasive and can be done in the privacy of your home. My patients have received outstanding results after following these simple directions and protocols. I will explain the exact details for each procedure in Chapter Seventeen: Cleansing Protocals. I have very successfully incorporated these activities to help patients control their own destinies, and not be like a puppet on strings.

CLEANSING PROTOCOLS

Colonic

A healthy colon is essential to a healthy body. Conventional diets comprised of refined, processed foods, high in saturated fats and low in fiber contribute to many problems associated with the large intestine. The elimination of undigested food material and other waste products are as important as the digestion and assimilation of food stuffs. Waste material allowed to remain stagnant in the colon results in decomposition of these substances and increased bacteria and their toxins.

The colon contains the largest concentration of bacteria in the body. These bacteria provide important functions such as the synthesis of folic acid, B-vitamins and vitamin K from foods. Bacillus coli and acidophilus comprise the majority of the healthy bacteria in the colon along with small numbers of other disease producing bacteria. Waste material permitted to stagnate alters the proportion of healthy bacteria to disease producing bacteria, allowing the potential for disease to exist. These bacteria decompose proteins and carbohydrates resulting in the production of toxins. Some of the toxins are thought to be absorbed and may be a potential source of disease elsewhere in the body. The purpose of the colon as an eliminative organ is to remove this waste material by mass muscular contraction called peristalsis. Colon hydrotherapy provides therapeutic improvement of muscular tone, facilitating peristalsis and benefiting the atonic (sluggish) colon. The effects of a stagnant colon can be manifested in the form of constipation, halitosis (bad breath), skin blemishes, headaches, low back pain and lack of energy.

Liver/Gallbladder Flush

Reasons for a Liver Flush:

- Blood sugar fluctuations
- Chemical sensitivities
- Cholesterol above 225
- Digestion discomfort
- Dizziness and/or the "shakes"
- Dry tongue and mouth
- Elevated liver enzymes
- Chronic constipation
- Extreme fatigue
- Eye floaters
- Female with tender breasts and heavy menstrual flow
- Dry hair and hair loss
- Headaches
- Mental problems/depression
- Muscle and bone pain
- Nails that peel or break
- Pain in the right side of abdomen
- Breathing distress
- Skin eruptions, moles, birth marks that are growing, acne, psoriasis

- ⬆ Susceptibility to infection
- ⬆ Unexplained weight gain and or tendency to gain weight easily

Coffee Enema

Now is the time I am going to really stretch you a bit. My wife, Deb, was diagnosed with dysplasia when she was about thirty years old. This would have been after our second child was born. One of the points we have learned is that cells can come and go on a cervical scraping, especially after having a child. We decided that what we were doing up until that point was not promoting optimal liver function on anyone in our families' lives. We made a total flip from consuming fried and processed foods, alcohol and soda to eating living, whole foods that did not burden our bodies with the addition of processed or toxic items.

We needed to be committed. There is a point I would like to reiterate and ask you: if Deb would have had the abnormal cells burned or cauterized, would we have been getting to the cause of the problem? No, of course not. To get to the cause, we needed to clean the machine.

After having a surgical procedure and when you are told by your doctor, "we got everything," do not get a false sense of security that you are normal. That statement pointedly speculates they got all the abnormal tissue and cells visible to their eyes at the time, but you need to know that an area in the body, which could be remotely involved, might still be creating the environment that allows more abnormal cells to appear.

I cringe when someone tells me this enormous mass of tissue was removed from their body, and they confidently look at me with the false belief that they are healed. I often learn that those individuals succumb to the same debilitating condition later on in life. No one took the time, either out of ignorance or denial of reality, to suggest that the patient might want to modify some area of their lifestyle. This is your life!

My wife didn't just stop at changing her diet. She was told that a coffee enema would benefit her overall health program, although, she really had never done enemas before, let alone coffee enemas. She would make a pot of organic coffee, using water filtered through an organic paper filter.

She self-administered regular coffee enemas for a year. The coffee enema physiologically works because the coffee is very aggravating to the system and the liver literally goes "berserk" when there is that much insult. Now, is the coffee enema something you have to do? Well, let me say this, it is nearly twenty-five years since my wife first started to make lifestyle changes. She has gone in for timely pap smears and other female procedures without ever having an abnormal report. She will do coffee enemas several times a year now, but doing them frequetly is not important because she does not have the ingested toxic overload. We also get regular colonic irrigation, at least two times a year. And we do not willingly put any "outside in" toxins into our bodies.

Juicing

I am a believer in preventive maintenance. To me that means your life is geared to promote life versus sickness treatment. It is very apparent to me that most new patients who enter my office have abused their body by over eating toxic foods including pastries, sodas, cookies, donuts, chips, French fries and the list could go on. They do not exercise, and the thought of drinking anything else but coffee, tea, energy drinks or alcohol is not a part of their day planner.

If you have been diagnosed with cancer, then you will want to heed the following information. I encourage patients who have been diagnosed with cancer to drink at least one quart of fresh vegetable juice daily for a minimum of two months. The juice is to be made in eight-ounce increments and consumed immediately. I suggest the following items in the recipe: carrot, beet, ginger (a small piece), sweet apple, parsley, celery and cucumber. I recommend one tablespoon of organic green food and one tablespoon of organic flax powder, with five drops of dandelion root or Livco® from Standard Process Labs. You can also use turmeric instead of ginger in the juice or add it to your mixed green salad. Turmeric is an anti-tumor food. Please check the ingredients in the green food and avoid any with artificial sweeteners. This combination will assist the body in purifying itself and will also significantly assist in the alkalizing process of the system. Your goal is a saliva pH that is purple on the nitrizine paper, indicating an alkaline pH. Acid promotes cancer and alkaline promotes life. We live in a society and have diets that are acid in nature.

JUST TELL ME WHAT TO DO

- Cleansing is not about taking or doing something; cleansing is about changing your mindset from the thought pattern that you can eat with reckless abandonment and your body will just deal with it. That thinking and lifestyle pattern will result in health breakdown.

- Focus on drinking water from a pure source. Minimize the amount of fluids that have preservatives and sweeteners. Your liver has to process any unused chemical. The more you put in, the harder the organs of detoxification have to work.

- My primary suggestion to you would be to evaluate what you are putting into your body before you attempt to alter the chemistry for it to release what is in it. Your body physiologically may not be able to release accumulated toxins without distress.

- Your best mode of detoxification would be to avoid putting sugar, trans fat, prescription and over-the-counter medications, which are very potent, into your body. These substances are the primary causes of your toxic response.

- Focus on organic whole foods, especially raw veggies, i.e., broccoli, cabbage, cauliflower and Brussels sprouts, along with apples, beets and carrots. See the Page Diet in Chapter Twenty

NOTES_____

_____

_____

_____

_____

_____

_____

_____

7

Fuel the Thyroid to Keep the Body Going

The thyroid is often an overlooked gland in its role in the big picture of female health patterns. I am not sure how many health providers really understand its role in the daily performance of female health. I have many female patients whose entire hormonal puzzle is resolved by adding iodine and tyrosine; which you will learn about later.

A challenge you are confronted with as a patient today is that there seems to be a specialist for every system in the body. This may not seem obvious to you, but you can suffer with chronic dry skin, morning headaches that wear off as the day goes on, elevated cholesterol, depression and constipation if the thyroid is not fed the right food. If you have any of these symptoms, you might visit a dermatologist for your skin, a pain management specialist for your pain, an internist for your cholesterol, a gastroenterologist for your colon and a psychiatrist for your depression.

Do you know that it is common for females, both young and old, to visit a healthcare provider for depression? A good percent of the time the patient can be at the office with an undetected sub-clinical thyroid problem with serum blood testing that references within normal values. Two significant items that feed the thyroid to make thyroid hormone are Tyrosine (an amino acid or protein building block) and iodine which are often deficient in patients who have depression. Tyrosine is specific for helping individuals with depression.

I have seen a recent overabundance of very young ladies in their teens and early twenties who come to my office and who are taking not only one antidepressant but, often times, two of these psycho-sensitive medications. What appears to be the indiscriminate distribution of these emotionally-addictive drugs is what alarms me. Do you know that the side effects of these prescriptions include a risk of suicide during the first twenty-four to thirty-six hours of starting this medication? Are you aware that suicide is the third leading cause of death in teens?

The pattern for this breakdown of physiology resulting in emotional burnout often occurs right from the initial onset of birth. If a child is bottle fed versus breast fed with soy-based formula from the beginning of their lives, they are headed for potential challenges in their later years. Do you remember having growing pains when you were growing up? Did you experience pain on the front of your knee? Growing pains are a very common body signal for a youngster experiencing low thyroid function. How could that be? The soy found in baby formula is an anti-thyroid food. Children, who are not breast fed, are more than likely consuming food that impairs thyroid function from the beginning of life!! I have a number of very young patients who have been diagnosed with a sub par functioning thyroid gland.

I have found that many young women today appear to have an issue with depression because of their food choices. The current generation of young adults was raised by parents who were exposed to convenience foods in their early lives. This means that today's moms ate fries and chicken nuggets plus an array of convenience foods during their formative years and have since had babies who have now grown up and are in their late teens and early twenties. Convenience and fast food is fried in or is overloaded with unhealthy oils that do not make good hormone precursors. The thyroid gland, like other glands in the endocrine system, counts on healthy oil as a basis to make the precious hormone keys for the body to function.

"Dr. Bob," you might ask, "Why do you think we are having more issues with a low thyroid at such a young age?" My answer is a couple of logical possibilities, but first a question for you. Why are so many kids and adults diagnosed with ADHD, pain syndromes, heart and hormonal issues? The answer for both of these questions is primarily, poor fat metabolism. Food today is over-processed without enough proper minerals and vitamins remaining intact. This creates a state of poor sources of ingredients necessary to complete the metabolism of the food you eat. Soy, as I mentioned earlier, is in what appears to be nearly everything and depletes one of the key players, zinc, along with others.

The biggest issue I see with the thyroid, since it is so significant in the hormonal system, is that not enough iodine is being consumed. Also, many professionals appear to be focused on carbohydrates versus protein, and if protein is consumed it is some type of processed wanna-be meat. Do you ever wonder what is really in chicken nuggets, deli meats and sausage? Protein from a qualified, natural whole source is needed for L-Tyrosine.

Also, we are living in a culture where fat phobia is rampant. The public has been so focused on the low-fat diet that getting a drop of good oil to pass the lips of a good percent of the population is tougher than pulling teeth. The media has the general population believing that all oil is bad, so they now primarily eat low-fat, high-carbohydrate foods. Consequently, the thyroid does not have the proper oil it needs. When the thyroid is unable to function properly, it causes the body to run on low with no energy, and the system is pulling along. You will ultimately gain weight. To correct this pattern, all you need to eat is whole food with a source of protein and minerals.

In Chapter Sixteen: Reversing Unhealthy Patterns, I discuss how significant the thyroid is for the big picture of preventing destructive patterns that often result in cancer somewhere in the body, especially the breasts. I would like to explain to you in very simple terms how the thyroid operates. Thyroid function is significant for normal bowel movements, and it is an indicator of iodine sufficiency. It seems logical to assume that if the thyroid does not have enough iodine, the ovaries do not have enough. Therefore, you could prevent female hormone issues by considering the function of the thyroid gland.

Your thyroid gland is a small mass of tissue, normally weighing less than one ounce, located in the front of the neck. It is made up of two halves, called lobes that lie along the windpipe (trachea) and are joined together by a narrow band of thyroid tissue, known as the isthmus. (See the drawing in Chapter One.).

The thyroid is situated just below your "Adams apple," or larynx. During development (inside the womb), the thyroid gland originates in the back of the tongue, but it normally migrates to the front of the neck before birth. Sometimes it fails to migrate properly and is located high in the neck or even in the back of the tongue (lingual thyroid), which is very rare. At other times it may migrate too far and end up in the chest, which is also rare.

The function of the thyroid gland is to take iodine, found in many foods, and convert it into thyroid hormones, thyroxine (T4) and triiodothyronine (T3).Thyroid tissue cells combine iodine and the amino acid, tyrosine, to make T3 and T4. T3 and T4 are then released into the blood stream and are transported throughout the body where they control metabolism (conversion of oxygen and calories to energy). Every cell in the body depends upon thyroid hormones for regulation of their metabolism. The normal thyroid gland produces about 80 percent T4 and about 20 percent T3; however, T3 possesses about four times the hormone "strength" as T4.

The thyroid gland is under the control of the pituitary gland, a small gland the size of a peanut at the base of the brain. When the level of thyroid hormones drops too low, the pituitary gland produces Thyroid Stimulating Hormone (TSH) which stimulates the thyroid gland to produce more hormones. Under the influence of TSH, the thyroid will manufacture and secrete T3 and T4, thereby raising their blood levels. The pituitary senses this and responds by decreasing its TSH production. Imagine the thyroid gland as a furnace and the pituitary gland as the thermostat. Thyroid hormones are like heat. When the heat gets back to the thermostat, it turns the thermostat off. As the room cools (the thyroid hormone levels drop), the thermostat turns back on (TSH increases) and the furnace produces more heat (thyroid hormones).

The pituitary gland, as discussed earlier, is regulated by the hypothalamus. The hypothalamus is part of the brain and produces TSH Releasing Hormone (TRH) which tells the pituitary gland to stimulate the thyroid gland (release TSH). One might imagine the hypothalamus as the person who regulates the thermostat, since it tells the pituitary gland at what level the thyroid should be set.

When patients come into the office and we do their blood tests, I have noticed that more than half of them have less than a level of 2 on their TSH serum levels. I suspect that the reason is the pituitary, like the rest of the body, also needs nutrients to survive. We use whole food Cataplex E® and Manganese®; or you could use a combined product called Vitamin E Manganese®. The particular product can be determined by tissue mineral analysis. This phenomenon is also common with patients who have stress in the adrenal gland, which is discussed in Chapter 8. I commonly see a minimal desire for sexual intimacy with individuals who also have a low TSH. This is consistent, and I believe that there must be a correlation with the physiologic burnout of the system.

There is also an epidemic of "iodine phobia" where physicians have not been encouraging supplementation with an organic source of iodine. Table salt has been a tool used to incorporate iodine into the masses that has not really been the best quality source of iodine. Commercial grade sodium chloride also has anti-caking constituents, including aluminum and dextrose (sugar), so the table salt will flow uninterrupted.

The public today not only has a fat phobia, they also have a salt phobia. Patients have been told to avoid salt because it raises blood pressure. I have found that salt may raise blood pressure in about five percent of the patients (and mind you, that is sodium chloride, the salt the masses consume). I do not consume commercial grade table salt.

What I really see what raises blood pressure is the huge appetite for sweets. Sugar raises the insulin level in the body and stresses the adrenal gland, raising blood pressure. Your body compensates with increased sodium retention. Increased sodium retention creates more water withholding. I also see blood pressure elevation in patients who do not drink enough water. When someone does not drink enough water, the blood gets thicker and more concentrated, restricting its flow, probably just the opposite of what you may think. Drink *at least* one quart of pure water daily.

I encourage Celtic Sea Salt® which is harvested from the Northern coast of France. Nothing has been added to it. The granules come from the open rock surface where the salt has evaporated from ocean water. It should be called Celtic Sea

Minerals instead of Sea Salt. Celtic Sea Salt® it is an excellent source of minerals and I encourage our patients to use it liberally.

Nearly every female patient that enters my office today is on thyroid medication of some sort. It can be the standard Synthroid or Armour Thyroid. Thyroid hormone, like insulin, from a cow or outside source does not repair the gland; in this case the thyroid.

I have observed some interesting issues with thyroid testing. I commonly find a low TSH in most patients with thyroid symptoms. I support the body with whole food supplements from Standard Process called Neuroplex®, Hypothalmex® and/or Pituitrophin PMG®. These are organ extracts and protomorphogens (a proprietary system creating a product with characteristics to assist the body to restore cell function, abbreviated as PMG) and are from animal sources. They feed the organs nutrients and assist in the restoration of cell metabolism.

I look to see if my patients have the following symptoms when doing a serum assessment of their thyroid. I generally look for at least six symptoms in conjunction with the blood tests that have a predetermined range.

Increase in weight	Decrease in appetite	Fatigue easily
Ringing in ears	Sleepy during day	Sensitive to cold
Dry or scaly skin	Constipation	Mental sluggishness
Hair coarse, falls out	Reduced initiative	Impaired hearing
Slow pulse, below 72	Frequency of urination	

Other body signals include: a morning headache that wears off as the day goes on, thinning of the outer eyebrows and the hair on the side of the legs, elevated cholesterol, wide-spaced teeth, cold hands and feet, dry skin and growing pains (as previously discussed) in kids.

What I have found, as noted above, is that we have three main serum levels to look at. I want to briefly discuss my parameters. If the TSH is less than 2, I support Pituitary gland function. If the TSH is greater that 2 but less than 10, I support the Thyroid gland with a protein-sourced product called Thyrotrophin PMG®. I also make sure the patient is consuming a source of Essential Fatty Acids, including the Omega 3 and 6 fats. Often I will supplement the patient with a product that supports the RNA and DNA template. I use a product called Ribonucleic Acid® from the same source as the other items I have mentioned thus far. It may take six months to two years before you see changes in the blood serum levels.

I also like to assess the T3 and T4 levels. Generally, I like to see both of those numbers above the midline as I observe the testing reference range from the lab. If the values are at the mid point or less, I generally focus on supplementing with an organic source of iodine. I use Prolamine Iodine® and Iodomere® or Cataplex F® tablets . Go slow with the iodine; you may notice a skin rash, metalic taste in your mouth, and/or pain over the eyes. I also like to supplement with a source of Tyrosine and a full spectrum amino acid. I normally use a product called Protefood® or Nutrimere® from Standard Process. There are many fine professional companies that make excellent individual sources of Tyrosine.

A point of reference: taking any supplement whether it is natural or synthetic can interfere with some medications, and some individuals have symptoms which appear to indicate they are sensitive to iodine. Your body is adapting to the release of the toxic effects of fluorine, chlorine and bromine that are being displaced by iodine. These symptoms will go away in a few days. Patients on heart medication may notice heart beat alterations with iodine. Always talk to a knowledgeable healthcare professional. Do not attempt to take large doses of iodine on your own when you are taking Amiodarone, Pacerone, or Cardarone.

Japanese women, who have a track record of minimal menopause symptoms or hot flashes, consume up to 12mg of iodine a day in their food, normally from fish and sea vegetables. I know first hand, from spending extended time in Japan, that sea vegetables and fresh marine life are a major source of their staple. The Japanese eat as a family and you don't see them eating out at fast food chains like we do in our Western Culture. Their markets are overflowing with fresh fish that is available daily.

The really critical lab value that is a concern is when the T4 is elevated in relation to the T3. That is a flag to me that the T4 is not converting over to T3. This is usually a sign that the patient may have one of two issues to deal with: stress with associated high cortisol levels and high estrogen. Both of these characteristics can impair thyroid hormone production. Elevated estrogen interrupts the production of thyroid hormone and creates a loop of negative feedback production that results in the thyroid not functioning. With the bowels and liver not operating at one-hundred percent, the estrogen builds up, and we have stagnation with estrogen dominance; a tough cycle to break.

I like to see the patient's dietary journal to make sure they are eating adequate protein. Often times, females do not consume enough protein, i.e., chicken, turkey and periodic red meat. I suggest that my patients take a full-spectrum protein supplement containing all the essential amino acid building blocks for protein called, Protefood® (at least one a day) to provide the amino acids for liver detoxification. You can use the thyroid hormone levels to gauge hormonal health when you use a skilled, experienced healthcare provider in your team of professionals.

I have encouraged many women to learn to say, "I cannot say yes" to many of their commitments that put them on overload. They are politely saying, "No." Ladies, for you to get to the level of health that you desire, you more than likely will have to assess your commitments to give your body an opportunity to reset itself and achieve a normal restful status.

I have patients monitor their armpit temperature while they are following the supplement protocol determined by the serum blood test. An important factor is that they have at least six symptoms from the list of low thyroid body signals (see Chapter Seven).

The thyroid can also be monitored by observing the results of mineral tissue hair analysis; more about that in Chapter Fifteen on Testing. Monitoring includes analyzing the ratios between mineral levels. A common sub-par thyroid pattern would include a calcium level that is proportionately higher than potassium levels; the ratio is normally 4:1. There are many tools that can be used to assess the function of your Thyroid. Your goal is to wake up without a headache, have awesome, smooth skin, regular bowel movements, a vibrant attitude and emotional state and cholesterol at the 200 level without medication or herbs. That would surely indicate you are going in the right direction, and on the way to optimal, whole-body health, with a finely stoked thyroid gland.

JUST TELL ME WHAT TO DO!!

- If you have the body signals described above, take your armpit or axillary temperature as discussed in the Chapter Three on Progesterone. If you have cold hands and feet, that would be a strong indicator that you may, in fact, have a sub-par functioning thyroid gland.

- If your temperature is less than 97.8°F, I would recommend locating a healthcare provider that understands assessing the serum blood thyroid values as I discussed above. You would want to consult with that individual and follow the protocol I mentioned for several months, then be retested. Do not go off your medications without being under the direct supervision of a qualified professional.

- I would not take a supplement protocol until you have had either the serum blood analysis and/or hair analysis, preferably both to have a base line to establish the criteria for supplementation.

- A hair analysis may be of value to determine the state of your mineral tissue levels of calcium and potassium. You would treat accordingly from the lab report results. See the Chapter Fifteen on Testing.

- Observe how your body signals change over time, that, in conjunction with your other testing, will help plot the course for your female hormonal stabilization.

- You may want to get a shower de-chlorinator. Chlorine is toxic to the thyroid. I encourage our patients to replace their standard, shower head with one that takes out chlorine. You can smell the difference with a decreased amount of chlorine in your shower stall air. I have located a shower head that has a long life and does not need the content or filter replaced because you backwash the material from the filter.

NOTES_____

_____
_____
_____
_____
_____
_____
_____
_____

Patient Testimony:

"I had various hormonal issues before making the lifestyle changes recommended by Dr. DeMaria. I had PMS, headaches for several days prior to my cycle and very tender breasts. I took Nsaids for cramping and headaches. Following Dr. Bob's suggestions, I eliminated all trans fats, reduced sugar, focused on lean meats and veggies and cut out most dairy.

Since making these lifestyle modifications I virtually have no PMS and only minimal cramping. My cycles are very regular!" **Laura Meyer**

Portions of this information were cited from: Endocrine Web http://www.endocrineweb.com/hypo1.html

8

Supporting the Adrenal Glands

The Adrenal Glands are a pair of glands located on top of your kidneys. They are situated right around the area where you're low and mid back areas would meet. They are by far the most overlooked pair of significant tissues for your overall, long-term, female health. The adrenal gland is similar to a fuel pump and your thyroid would be like the gas pedal. The two work together in unison with the pancreas, liver, and of course, the rest of the body.

When I read about the adrenal glands they always seem to refer to the story about the fire, and how you respond. The adrenal glands are the organs that let you "high tail" it out of a situation when you need to get going. They create the response in the body thart speeds up the heart, gets the muscles the fuel they need, and all the other details to "get out of town." Today, in our fast-paced, cell phone, double-eared, "Blue Toothed" connection office in the vehicle society, our adrenal glands are exhausted from trying to keep up, constantly putting out all the little-big fires.

What most don't realize is that the adrenal glands are designed as a part of your long-term, back-up hormonal replacement part system. As time and technology move on, I believe the masses will put as much energy into keeping their adrenals healthy as they do in maintaining their pearly white smile and keeping their blood vessels clear. The adrenal glands are a part of a sophisticated system of interchangeable related steroid chemicals necessary for life. Steroids used in this context would be the basic building blocks for the sex hormones in the body.

Below is a chart with names that I don't expect you to pronounce, but I want you to see the maze. You will see advertisements telling you if you consume this pill you will lose weight, or if you take this pill your muscles will get big, or ladies if you take and rub this cream, you will have an increased desire to have sex, your bones will get strong and you won't have heart issues. It all starts with cholesterol, the designated "bad boy" in health. Cholesterol is not good or bad. It is necessary and does its job. Unfortunately for some, the job it is doing requires a transport system that takes it to the site of inflammation.

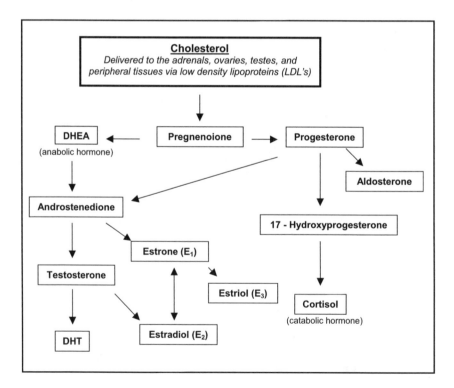

Do you see how it all starts with Cholesterol? Cholesterol has the potential to be an important end product for our discussion: estrogen, progesterone and cortisol. The big craze now is Vitamin D. You're reading in the magazines to take your D so you don't break a bone. I would suggest you go in the sun every day. Avoid hiding from the sun. Make sure you take some extra flax oil and calcium for the sun to have something to work with. The sun converts the cholesterol in your skin to Vitamin D. Do you want to help your body to lower your cholesterol? Then get in the sun. Also watch what you are putting on your skin to block out the rays. If you see the ingredient Sodium-lauryl-Sulfate, a known carcinogen, put it down. Whatever you put on your skin will ultimately enter the body. Be aware and cautious, reading all the ingredients. Lotions and gels will be processed by the body and can create cysts!! Makes you wonder what is causing cancer anyway, the lotion or the sun? What you put on your skin is absorbed into your body, and your liver has to work on getting it out.

The adrenal gland has two functional portions to it. The inner part is called the medulla and the outer part is the cortex. I would like to focus on the cortex. Situated along the perimeter of the adrenal gland, the adrenal cortex mediates the stress response through the production of mineral corticoids (for mineral regulation) and glucocorticoids (for sugar metabolism and cortisone). It is also a secondary site of androgen (sex hormone) synthesis.

Androgen can be defined as the generic term for any natural or synthetic compound, usually a steroid hormone, that stimulates or controls the development and maintenance of masculine characteristics in humans by binding to androgen receptors. This includes the activity of the accessory male sex organs and development of male secondary sex characteristics.

Androgens, which were first discovered in 1936, are also called androgenic hormones or testoids. Androgens are also the original anabolic steriods. They are also the precursor of all estrogens, the female sex hormones. The primary and most well-known androgen is testosterone; a critical point in our discussion for long-term, female health and why menopausal women should not have to deal with hormone issues.

The adrenal glands, just like the other glands in your body, need quality food for their job description to be fulfilled. A HUGE point for all the hormone producing glands is they need oil from a quality source. I personally prefer an organic source of plant oils, especially the Omega 3 fats such as the precursor flax oil or a marine based oil product like tuna, salmon or other "fatty fish." I do not encourage farm raised fish. The low-fat diet has been a major obstacle for female health. Your body uses the oils as a basis for hormone production. Low fat means you are not getting the right ingredients. The focus on calories versus quality has created the foundation for poor female health.

Adrenal fatigue body signals are occurring in epidemic proportions. Most people that I talk with in my practice and throughout America have several common symptoms. I have provided a checklist to help you assess your own potential challenges with your adrenal function.

Adrenal Fatigue Checklist...
How many do you have?

- ☑ Difficulty getting up in the morning
- ☑ Continuing fatigue, not relieved by sleep and rest
- ☑ Lethargy, lack of energy to do normal daily activities
- ☐ Sugar cravings
- ☐ Salt cravings
- ☑ Allergies
- ☐ Digestion problems
- ☑ Increased effort needed for everyday tasks
- ☐ Decreased interest in sex
- ☐ Decreased ability to handle stress
- ☐ Increased time needed to recover from illness, injury or traumas
- ☐ Light-headed or dizzy when standing up quickly
- ☑ Low mood
- ☑ Less enjoyment or happiness with life

- ☐ Increased PMS
- ☐ Symptoms worsen if meals are skipped or inadequate
- ☑ Thoughts are less focused, brain fog
- ☑ Memory is poorer
- ☑ Decreased tolerance for stress, noise, disorder
- ☐ Don't really wake up until after 10:00 a.m.
- ☐ Afternoon low between 3:00 and 4:00 p.m.
- ☐ Feel better after supper
- ☐ Get a "second wind" in the evening and stay up late
- ☑ Decreased ability to get things done – less productive
- ☑ Have to keep moving – if I stop, I get tired
- ☑ Feeling overwhelmed by all that needs to be done

Factors leading to Adrenal Fatigue
How many do you have?

- ☐ White Sugar and White Flour Products
- ☐ Lack of relaxation
- ☐ Smoking
- ☐ Antacids
- ☐ Devitalized Food
- ☐ Unfulfilling Employment (dead-end jobs)
- ☐ Dead-End Relationships
- ☐ Surgery
- ☐ Junk Food
- ☐ Trans Fats/Rancid Fats
- ☐ Financial Stress
- ☐ Sedentary Lifestyle
- ☐ Excessive Exercise
- ☐ Death of a Loved One
- ☐ Alcoholism
- ☐ Toxins
- ☐ Poor Eating Habits
- ☐ Hormonal Imbalances
- ☐ Oral Contraceptives
- ☐ Stimulants

- ☐ Counterproductive Attitudes & Beliefs
- ☐ Conventional Hormone Replacement Therapy
- ☐ Non-Prescription Drugs
- ☐ Psychological Stress
- ☐ Persistent Fears
- ☐ Emotional Stress
- ☐ Lack of Sleep
- ☐ Being in Denial about Feelings
- ☐ Infection, Acute or Chronic
- ☐ Repeated Stresses
- ☐ Persistent Negative Stressors
- ☐ Fun or Enjoyment Deprivation
- ☐ Allergies
- ☐ Caffeine
- ☐ Prescription Drugs
- ☐ Marital Stress
- ☐ Repeated Traumas
- ☐ Workaholic

The situation I regularly see includes the following scenario: A life that starts on soy-based, high phyto-estrogen baby formula, then a childhood focused on snacks, processed and pre-made foods (macaroni and cheese and chicken nuggets). The teen years include soda, relentless cravings for chocolate and peanut butter candies, fatty-sourced, high trans-fat foods from the fast food venues, and some teens give in to either self-starvation or overeating. The teens progress quickly to young adulthood, eating very little fresh veggies and whole foods; the diet is devoid of health-promoting oil and concentrated on eating on the run at one of many local franchise restaurants. By this time, the list of prescription medications starts with an antidepressant, antihistamines and/or combinations of pain relievers and antihistamines. The young ladies start to have the beginnings of heavy menstrual flow, cysts on the breast, a possible cyst or two on the ovaries and cystic breast disease. The menstrual cycle is very painful and even debilitating, with a hormone-related headache at the end of the flow. This scenario quickly becomes the young lady sprinting into her late forties before she knows it. She may be one of the statistics for gallbladder, uterus and/or ovary removal and then comes the BIG question: WHAT DO I TAKE?

The adrenal glands are there to rescue you. A part of their job description is to be the back-up to provide enough hormones to carry you through all the cycles of your life. A common pattern I see in my practice is the onset of menses before the age of ten, which is often followed by a lifetime of tender breasts and heavy menstrual flow (caused by premenopause estrogen saturation) and concludes with challenges in menopause because the adrenal glands now cannot make enough estrogen to support the natural requirements necessary for optimal health.

The adrenal glands are designed to release whatever female hormone you may need. What generally happens is the patient is addicted to sugar. That passionate craving upsets the very sensitive balance of the production of hormones for sexual and bone and joint function.

When you consume sugar, your body needs to process it. The mechanism requires the adrenal gland to shift the focus of production to make glucocorticoids (mentioned above) to process the nutritionally devoid character of the sugar. Production of the mineral corticoids and sex hormones suffers. The patient with this history will come in and complain of their back going out easily, a loss of a desire to have sexual intimacy and pain syndromes like fibromyalgia.

Let me explain. The back goes out easily because your adrenals are not making the mineral corticoid to absorb adequate minerals. You need minerals for ligaments to be strong. Then you crave salt. You lose the desire for sex because the sex hormone portion of the adrenal cortex is focused on processing the sugar. Finally, you're in chronic pain, because the cortisone used for pain is also being used up to process the sugar.

You're not going to be a party to be around because you will have a multitude of symptoms related to what you eat. Pain will be with you twenty-four hours a day, seven days a week. The last thing you want is to have someone wanting to be with you sexually, and you will be craving sugar and salt because you are deficient in minerals. You will more than likely be advised to take an antidepressant because of the stress you are under. The real answer to your misery is to work on breaking the cycle.

If your adrenal glands are exhausted when you are in your twenties and thirties, what is going to happen when you are in your fifties and your body is now starving for estrogen? Where is it going to come from? Your ovaries are shutting down and the rest of your body is totally exhausted. Are you really going to want to take a synthetic hormone that is based from pregnant mare urine, trade marked as Premarin®?

I would like to talk you a bit about a loop I see. I purposely put the chemistry-like chart in this chapter because I needed you to see that cholesterol is a very big player in the scheme of things. Your body will make cholesterol if you don't eat enough of it. Cholesterol is literally in nearly every cell membrane of the body.

Cholesterol is not readily absorbed in water so it needs to be carried by—what I like to call a fire truck—lipoprotein. The fire truck that carries the cholesterol to the fire is called LDL; the one that returns it to the fire house is HDL. If you have recently had a blood test indicating "high cholesterol" and the well-meaning physician suggested a cholesterol-lowering drug, do you know that taking that drug is like shooting yourself in the foot? You're actually shooting the "fireman" and opening yourself up to a list of negative side effects associated with these medications.

The cholesterol is elevated because your brain has been notified you need more cholesterol to make the list of hormones on the maze. The questions you need to ask yourself are: what is the reason the cholesterol is in demand, and what is causing the fire? The answers, from my experience and looking at years of diet journals, are complex but correctable: sugar, trans fat or partially hydrogenated oil, dairy and the low fat diet. These items interfere with normal fat metabolism critical for optimal hormonal health. You will learn more about that in Chapter Twenty-two on Fat. I have written an entire book on this one subject alone, *Dr. Bob's Trans Fat Survival Guide,* which is available at www.DruglessDoctor.com.

Your adrenal glands need the cholesterol to do their job. Your consumption of sugar and refined foods create stress on the adrenal glands to modify production, and hence, you will have menstrual issues and eventually menopausal challenges.

JUST TELL ME WHAT TO DO

- A real key to long-term adrenal health is coordinating your life so you have time to rest. I know this may not be easy for some, but it will help in your long-term protocol. Sleep eight hours a night. No lights on. Limit your TV and computer time before bed. Cover the lights in your bedroom, i.e., the alarm clock, little lights on DVD's, VCR's and other electrical appliances.

- Sugar, by far, is one of the most detrimental items that affect your adrenal health. I would take up to nine Cataplex GTF® a day to help minimize the cravings for sugar. Gymnema® is an excellent herb that reduces the taste for sweet items, one to three daily.

- Focus on getting more protein into your diet. Protein helps your energy burning in the body to stabilize. You won't have those sugar highs and lows. Your system will burn muscle when it cannot get enough energy from poor carbohydrates. Limit protein to three to five ounces per serving so you do not get a compensatory insulin release, starting a cascade of cravings.

- Avoid sweet fruits especially bananas, raisins and grapes. Eat veggies as a snack with some nuts, like almonds, walnuts and sunflower seeds.

- If you crave salt, which is a common adrenal fatigue body signal, consume Celtic Sea Salt®.

- Do not put progesterone cream on your body once your adrenal gland is up to par. Do not take DHEA, it can throw your system off. You want to have your saliva assessed for DHEA and cortisol, and support the body with whole-food supplementation, herbal tonics and adaptaogens. You will need a skilled healthcare provider to assist you.

- You may want to have your blood pressure taken lying down, then standing up. Your blood pressure should not drop.

- Salvia progesterone and estrogen testing may assist you in your supplement protocol. I suggest using Drenamin® Drentatrphin PMG® and Adrenal Whole Dessicated®, depending on the severity of the condition. These whole food supplements support adrenal restoration.

- I recommend taking whole food Cataplex C®, anywhere from three to nine a day. Vitamin C is an integral component of adrenal health.

- I also recommend Cataplex B® for patients when their blood pressure is low. You will want to be monitored by an experienced healthcare provider.

Synthetic B vitamins may, in fact, aggravate the adrenals.

- You can monitor your progress by assessing your blood pressure.

- A hair analysis is also a useful tool to help you monitor you adrenal health. Commonly, I see low sodium and potassium when a patient has stressed adrenal function. Aluminum is often high when the adrenal glands are overworked.

NOTES_____

_____

_____

_____

_____

_____

_____

_____

_____

9
Strengthen the Frame and Structure

Osteoporosis

O steoporosis is a condition that is very commonly discussed today and one of the many frequent reasons that your medical healthcare provider will suggest hormone replacement therapy or some other type of prescription to stop the loss of bone. The approach of prescription medicine stops nature from doing its job, and in the long run, will actually create osteoporosis. Osteoporosis, simply put, is the loss of the structural density of bone. Think of it as washing your clothes so often that the brilliant colors you love on your favorite cotton blouse begin to slowly leave and then finally one day it is visibly faded.

The exact cause of osteoporosis is theoretically, not precisely, known by many physicians. The public has been positioned as players in the guessing game as to the cause of osteoporosis and has been told that you must take medication to stop it.

There are many reasons why it is prevalent that I am sure will make sense once I describe the possibilities. Not all women in America have osteoporosis. If it was at epidemic levels, then one and all would be diagnosed with it. Since all women do not have it, there must be a pattern that creates bone loss for those who do. If I can help you discover your pattern and then reverse it, we can stop it and manage it.

I can tell you that taking one of the new once-a-month, highly-promoted, celebrity-endorsed medications only tricks the body and does not get to the cause of the problem. These prescriptions are peddled on a premise of fear. Fear that if you do not take them you will wake up one day and be bent over with your eyes staring at your feet.

The medications that women are being told they need once every thirty days works by preventing a bone cell called an osteoclast from doing its job. You see an osteoclast's job description is to vacuum up bone cells that need to be recycled. It is something like the Pac-Man creature going around eating everything in sight. The whole mechanism is very controlled by the innate intelligence that controls the way the structural system maintains itself. Your body is in a constant state of transition of breakdown and repair. This occurs at the cellular level. It occurs gradually over time.

The real issue with these medications is they are not getting to the cause of the problem. The medications are giving the user a false sense of security, just like other medications that treat symptoms versus cause. Over time, using medications that interfere with the osteoclast's work results in old, fragile bone being present where there should be new, strong bones with vitality.

When someone currently on osteoporosis medication has bone density scans performed on various areas, it appears that there is structure, giving the false sense of security I was telling you about, but it is not normal for old bone to be present. Vertebrae can fracture when on osteoporosis medication. I am not suggesting that you stop your meds without making other lifestyle changes. You will want to talk to a healthcare provider that can monitor your progression.

When I see osteoporosis in a new patient, it looks like the bone has been washed out on x-ray. The outer margin, or rim, around the bone has what is called a "pencil thin cortex." This is a characteristic that I evaluate when I am assessing osteoporosis on patient films.

So I want you to think; why do natural fabric cotton clothes (bones) fade? Because you use them and there is relentless friction, plus wear and tear on the small fibers in the cloth, and sunlight also causes chemical changes in the dye, and of course, washing the fabric with detergent results in the color slowly leaving over time. The more you wear an outfit and wash it, the quicker you will replace it. But if you take care of the material, and wash it in the appropriate temperatures and use mild detergents it will last longer.

Osteoporosis is something that does not have to happen to a female when she hits the magic age of sixty-two or sixty-five. This may be new to you, but osteoporosis actually originates with habits that can start at the very beginning of life and the health of your birth mom is very significant.

I want to reiterate a point. We, and when I say we, I am including myself in the group, are constantly told by the media, who is fed information by the pharmaceutically-endorsed studies and free-lance writers who get paid to release information, that osteoporosis and other common chronic conditions are controlled by genetics, viruses and family characteristics. Writers specifically ask for what they need to have written by experts.

I have treated a substantial number of patients that have other family members with poor health, yet they (my patients), chose to make lifestyle changes. They started by eliminating the old family recipes from grandma and made a new, healthier life for themselves. There is more to it than being doomed if someone in your family has a condition that has been determined to be incurable.

I generally see signs of osteoporosis in new female patients in their late sixties or seventies. I normally do not see osteoporosis in patients in their forties or fifties unless they have smoked or have a history of obsessive sugar consumption. Smoking is an addiction that is serious. Smoking depletes the body of minerals and slows the healing of bone structures. Not all women I treat have osteoporosis.

I have noted that it is common to see osteoporosis in females who have considerable dental work visible on the lateral cervical or neck x-rays. My observation of this dental finding, in correlation with reviewing blood serum studies and attending post-graduate level training, suggests that there is a common abnormal pattern of having an altered serum level of two minerals. I will find elevated phosphorus levels along with low calcium in these same individuals. Generally, there should be, from a functional nutritional evaluation, parameters of ten parts of serum calcium to four parts serum phosphorous.

When you experience elevated phosphorous in the body, it is balanced by calcium. Consuming items such as grains and soda pop with a high phosphorous content can create an environment where the body slowly loses calcium. Phosphorous can also be increased when the body is using muscle for a fuel source because the carbohydrate fuel mechanism is not functioning properly.

Phosphorus is elevated in the serum and hair tissue analysis in patients who are burning muscle for fuel versus glucose or blood sugar. When patients are exposed to this information, they understand why their faulty eating patterns based on refined grains and pastries have been a part of their dilemma. Breads and pastas are regular items in the diet histories of patients who have osteoporosis.

There basically appears to be two types of individuals today. Those who are determined and very concerned about what they eat, and others who have either no regard or feel they are past the point of no return. Patients who change their lifestyle upon beginning natural healthcare management, never develop osteoporosis and other issues commonly accepted as normal in our media-driven society. My patients are reaping the benefits of being counter-culture by not following fads such as the low-fat, high-carbohydrate diet. Just because you may read something from a reputable institution does not mean it is accurate.

There have been many reports and headlines in the *Wall Street Journal* suggesting less than honorable details of the results of drug testing. In other words, the companies reporting information on new prescription medications were lying. I always like to chuckle when a representative of the pharmaceutical community, who does not understand natural care, asks me for "documented studies." I often respond that they can be found in the same study that said the XXXX drug you suggested was safe. They know full well that the medication caused harm. We are talking billions of dollars just on osteoporosis medications alone.

I have post World War II era patients in my clinical practice who, as adults, started care in 1978. They were in their forties and fifties and now are in their eighties and are spunky and moving around better than some of the new patients I see who are in their fifties and sixties. They came from a whole different generation of food and activity.

I was raised with food made and eaten at home. We only went to a fast food restaurant once or twice a year. Today, thirty percent of children between four and nineteen years old eat at a fast food establishment every day. You also need to take into consideration that the government feeds nearly thirty million kids everyday with food that leaves much to be desired.

I regularly manage patients and their relatives who are interested in making changes for their young families, creating lifestyle patterns that won't lead to osteoporosis. When a female has chronic, challenging menstrual cycles early in life, she will have other hormonal issues when she get older. It is always best to start a healthy lifestyle pattern right from the beginning.

It normally takes a 40 percent loss of bone structure to show up on an x-ray. The scale of osteoporosis scanning is based on findings of women in their thirties; knowing that, many women have the potential to manifest osteoporosis in America when they are compared to this scale. I look at several factors when assessing and suggesting a diagnosis of osteoporosis. Calcified rib cartilage is often evident in individuals with a pattern that results in bone loss later found in spinal vertebrae.

It has been suggested that estrogen therapy can slow osteoporosis. What if we can feed the body so it can process estrogen adequately on its own? I have seen from experience that improper food choices are one of the major reasons there is an osteoporosis epidemic. The body has a challenge making hormones when one does not supply the proper ingredients or eats nutritionally inadequate foods that are unable to create the proper supply of estrogen. Estrogen (in natural or synthetic forms from outside sources) in a compromised, functioning hormone system is not often properly processed by the liver. The liver is a very significant player in the process of hormone metabolism.

The human body has the potential to make estrogen from several sources. Feeding the body whole foods is one of the better ways to maintain adequate estrogen levels in the post-menopausal state. The adrenal glands and ovaries are also two of the major secondary post-menopausal sources of estrogen.

When a new patient with osteoporosis comes into the office, she needs to realize that she has developed a lifetime of eating and exercise patterns that created the condition of mineral loss which resulted in her physical condition. In order to see results, you have to come to the understanding that what you have done to your body up to this point in your life is the reason you are the way you are.

To get what you have never had before you must do something you have never done before. The three S's, Sugar, Soda and Stress are by far the leading factors leading to osteoporosis. Lack of activity is also a very key reason we nearly have an osteoporosis epidemic. Food groups that are acid, like meat, cheeses and grains will create an acid environment.

An acid ash diet promotes osteoporosis. Look at the p-H based food chart in the Appendix, focus on balancing and eating enough servings of the alkaline food group, especially when you eat acid ash based food groups.

The protective physiology of the body that occurs when the acidic quality of sugar is consumed results in minerals being forced out of their normal job description to neutralize the affects of the sweet crystals. Guess which area of the body is your mineral reservoir? You guessed it; the bones. Your body will have to take minerals from somewhere, very often it is your skeletal system and also your teeth.

Soda has an ingredient in it by the name of phosphoric acid which creates the effervescent bubbles found in your favorite beverage. Phosphoric acid leaches calcium out of the body. I would like you to start observing the teeth of our youth who smile with what looks like mottled or discolored teeth, or teeth with uneven whiteness; they are often heavy soda drinkers. The average American consumes over fifty gallons a year.

I also know that the stress of everyday living can create the redistribution of tissue calcium. I will often complete a tissue mineral analysis from a patient's hair sample from the nape of their neck. In reviewing the analysis it is often noted by the lab that the patient has plenty of calcium; it is just in the wrong places in the body. Someone who has stress can have an adaptive response with calcium depositing in the hair versus being what we call "bio-available" or "for use." The calcium is not ionizable. Stress can also elevate cortisol, a hormone from the adrenal gland. Elevated cortisol, either naturally or from medication, has a calcium-depleting effect. You may want to have a mineral tissue analysis completed to see what your levels are. It is a great non-invasive procedure that can actually give you a road map for your future.

Mineral tissue analysis, unlike serum calcium, give you a snapshot of what your past has been. It is also a pattern of what your future may hold. Blood serum calcium can fluctuate quickly because your body is constantly pursuing equilibrium. Your homeostasis balance for minerals will result in robbing Peter to pay Paul.

One of the visible body signals of stress that I commonly see are cold sore blisters on the lip. I always see them in individuals who are going through personal challenges. They nearly always have chronic calcium body signals, i.e., leg cramps, menstrual cramps, cold hands and feet, thick dry flaky skin, poison ivy and gray or white hair. The gray or white hair is also a sign of poor calcium body metabolism.

Calcium helps glue cell membranes together. When you run low on calcium, cell membrane defense mechanisms break down, and viruses are given the chance to move in between the cell membrane gaps, and you have herpes simplex on the lip. Herpes blisters on the lip are quite common in individuals who have financial distress, marital and other personal issues. Also, patients with blood type A seem to have more digestive distress with poor calcium absorption.

Your body converts the cholesterol in your skin to vitamin D. Vitamin D increases the demand of calcium absorption in the small intestine. Think of it this way. Being in the sun will help lower your cholesterol which is very good. If you do spend a lot of time in the sun, make sure you eat enough calcium-based foods, such as the cruciferous veggies including broccoli, cabbage and cauliflower, along with sesame seeds and almonds. A daily dose of sunshine does the body good. It creates calcium movement.

I see this calcium-depleting phenomenon a lot in "snow-birds" from the North that go to the sunny climates during the winter. They will often come home with a cold sore on their lip or lips, and more than that, they will have symptoms of a cold. I am bringing this up primarily because if you are eating foods with sugar or a high protein diet, which is an acid-producing ash or acid-residue diet, you will have a tendency to get cold sores when you are in the sun or stressed. You are living in a state of calcium depletion. You also have the tendency to be a candidate for osteoporosis. An ounce of prevention is worth a pound of cure.

There is a phenomenon that occurs in the body, and I will be easy on you with the words, called the piezoelectric effect. This is the response in the body where the stress placed on the supporting bone from gravity resistance pressure results in calcium being deposited to the points of weight bearing. If someone does not have weight bearing or resistance exercise on a regular daily basis, I can almost guarantee they will have some structural breakdown.

The body works just the opposite of a cotton shirt that gets washed out. The more gradual stress you place on a structure like bone, the stronger it gets. This is a very significant point for you to grasp.

Have you ever gone snorkeling or seen pictures of under water vegetation? Think of your spinal structures as sea coral. If you are a part of the coral reef facing the shore there will be very little resistance splashing on it from the ocean. On the other hand, if the coral is facing the open sea, with strong currents and the resistance of the water forcing itself on the coral reef and small structures, it will have a radiance of brilliant colors, often seen on beautiful post cards. The dazzling colors are there in much the same way that calcium is placed on the spinal vertebrae, hips and other weight-bearing structures. Sitting on the couch is very similar to the coral facing the bay side. You would do your body a favor by getting out and moving.

I have noticed, probably like many of you, typical western children are rarely outdoors any more. When my wife and I ride our bikes, we just do not see kids playing. I am sure many of you reading this can remember going outside to play first thing in the morning and not coming home till dusk, exhausted from playing with your friends. If you are in the shape you are in now, and I am not meddling, just questioning, what will happen to the current generation thirty or forty years from now? They do not play and/or run outside, creating a long-term pattern of exercise.

The children in our culture, as one attorney friend of mine said, do not even have to learn the skill of negotiation any more. All their activities are organized with referees and coaches telling them what to do. You can find an organized activity for nearly any event desired.

Electronic play toys have become the replacement for TV. Children used to have small game toys that distracted them, now it is to the point, as I just saw at a local restaurant, a small child playing games on his mom's cell phone.

I suggest that as a top priority you become more active. You need an exercise to get the heart pumping oxygen, such as riding a bike, jogging, roller blading, rowing or jumping on a mini-trampoline; any activity to get the lungs blowing off the extra acid. The lungs are an organ that helps stabilize pH or the acid and alkaline levels. I recommend strength training combined with aerobic activity as a start in improving your overall health.

I am NOT talking about water aerobics by the way. I am not suggesting water exercise is a poor choice, it is more appropriate for mobilization than it is for structural strength. I would also take your water exercise one step further, by the way. Chlorine depletes the body of sodium, so I would supplement my diet with a quality mineral supplement to replenish the sodium (not sodium chloride found in commercial table salt). Sodium is needed in the body for many reactions. If you are stiff and sore, you may need sodium, according to Donald Le Pore, author of *The Ultimate Healing System*. I encourage my patients to use Celtic Sea Salt® liberally.

The thyroid plays a huge role in the osteoporosis puzzle. Being low in thyroid is a very common condition today. It is estimated that one-third of the world's population is low in thyroid. The public in our country have a very strong tendency to not consume enough iodine. Taking salt with iodine added to it, by the way, does not guarantee you will achieve optimal iodine levels. When you have a low thyroid count in America, you are normally prescribed a thyroid medication by a conventional western medical practitioner. This medication does not consider hormones in the body to mobilize calcium.

The thyroid gland and its very close neighbor the para-thyroid are the major players. Between the two glands, they virtually control calcium movement in the body. One of the warnings on thyroid medication is not to take it long term or it will result in bony re-absorption, thereby reducing bone mineral density, especially in post menopausal women. This may result in increased excretion of calcium and phosphorus from the body.

You are advised, according to the label, to take the least amount to get the desired effect. So, as far out as this may sound, it is possible that the thyroid medication you have been on for years may be the primary single cause of your OSTEOPOROSIS. You can check this out yourself on the internet by doing a search on "thyroid medication. Synthroid is a common source. It is actually quite frightening. I am not telling you to get off your medication. This is a process that needs professional assistance with a skilled healthcare provider familiar with natural, drugless therapies.

Hot flashes are one of the significant reasons women are on hormone replacement therapy. What I would like you to be aware of is this. Are you ready? One of the primary causes of hot flashes is a low functioning thyroid gland, with or without medicinal support. So, if you are taking thyroid medication, you can lose bone long term and still have hot flashes. The thyroid medication is really not restoring thyroid function in the first place. I have witnessed patients who present themselves to my office who are taking thyroid medication and have hot flashes. When treated appropriately, they are relieved of the hot flashes and able to discontinue the thyroid medication. It takes time and lifestyle modification. You have to feed the thyroid, which I talk about in detail in Chapter Seven: Fuel the Thyroid to Keep the Body Going.

One of the current medical protocols is to utilize anti-depressants as a symptomatic Band-Aid™ to relieve the symptoms of a hot flash. It was just recently released that these same antidepressants used for hot flashes can also have many negative side effects which include loss of bone density or osteoporosis.

So we are living in a Catch-22. My suggestion is to focus on the appropriate lifestyle changes that were mentioned previously which allow the body to function optimally without symptomatic treatment.

Thyroid issues can actually start very young. I bring this up because, as a Natural Healthcare provider, I have the opportunity to see patients of all ages. I have seen babies from a few hours old to patients over one hundred years of age. One very common thread I see in youngsters under ten, who may have initial body signals of a low thyroid, is a fever of an unknown cause.

Do you know what I have found to be one of the leading factors causing a fever? Not enough calcium. This occurs during several important physiologic times, i.e., when a child is teething and when they are ready to have a "growing spurt." There is a demand being placed on their own calcium reserve.

These same children often also have growing pains. I see growing pains a lot in children who have body signals of a low thyroid that is not functioning up to par. Probably the most common symptoms include cold hands and feet. Yes, children can have a low thyroid with an associated low body temperature. I have had children as new patients who have been on thyroid medication from very early in their lives, and some have even had their thyroid surgically removed.

The armpit temperature should be measured in the morning when they first get up, and used as a gauge to see how they are responding. I would also recommend the normal thyroid blood tests, to be evaluated by a healthcare provider who can assess the ranges, even if they are within a laboratory designation of normal. I would not necessarily want to see a child put on thyroid medication until a nutritional assessment was completed. A lot of time, stress can cause thyroid physiology problems.

If you remember having some of those symptoms when you were a child, chances are your body never got over it. You may have a calcium metabolism issue that more than likely started when you were very young.

I did when I was a child. I had growing pains and terrible discomfort in various joints in my body that hurt when I played ball. My parents took me to all types of doctors who treated the symptoms, not the cause. If you had growing pains as a kid, you will want to work hard on reversing some of your patterns that deplete the body of calcium; when your calcium reserve is under stress, then your thyroid will be stressed.

Let me tie a little of this together for you. If a child has a fever when their calcium is low, could that also result in a possible state of "fever" or "hot flash" in an adult? My experience says "yes." On observation of women with osteoporosis and hot flashes, it is revealed on hair analysis that calcium is present in their hair, but it is not available at the cellular level.

One of the areas most noticable affected by osteoporosis is the spine, since it has a bearing upon your posture. Therefore, if your head is in a forward position, it will put additional abnormal stress on your spine. Gravity is either working with or against you. A part of your long-term preventative maintenance would be to alter or change postural mechanics. Seek a skilled Chiropractor who would do your body real good. Check Chapter Ten: Communication Between the Brain and Tissue Cells regarding subluxation . You will want to do some of the exercises that I have described below.

Another key to your long-term prevention of osteoporosis is toning the tissues in your body. The patients I attract are tired of being on medications, and they realize that they are the captains of their own ships. I highly recommend that you exercise everyday. Let me tell you something, I know your pain. I see it everyday. I have patients that may be just like you. They are not happy with how they feel and look, butand this is a big BUT, no pun intended—they make an educated decision to change. It takes TIME. This is not an excuse, it is physiologic. It takes time.

If you are overweight and unhappy with how you look, the last place you want to go to is an exercise class with women in tights who have been working out for years. I suggest that you find an exercise class for beginners. They are around, you just need to seek and ask. Go to one of the classes that would best fit your time schedule and commit to it. Managing osteoporosis either medically or naturally is a process. It takes determination, discipline and effort. It can happen; I see it all the time. If it can occur for my patients, it can be a reality for you.

Managing osteoporosis requires a full-spectrum approach. I do not want you to have a false sense of security that taking a once-a-month pill is getting to the cause of the condition. I would encourage you to become proactive in your lifestyle. Do not become discouraged. It has taken time for your body to arrive at the state it is in, and it will take time to restore function. Start today. Look over the following suggestions. These are the same recommendations that I have used for the last thirty years with amazing results!

STEPS TO STRUCTURAL RESTORATION

- I would first suggest completing a food journal and assess how much sugar and soda you consume in a day. If you are a soda and sugar addict, I would encourage a whole food source of chromium which helps minimize those relentless urges to eat another piece. I recommend taking Cataplex GTF®, up to nine tablets daily, from Standard Process, a source of whole food chromium, until the craving for sugar subsides. Then, I would slowly reduce the chromium to a maintenance level of one or two daily. You want the cravings stopped. I also suggest an herb called

Gymnema®, one to three tablets daily. This herb works by reducing your taste for sweets. A tissue mineral analysis of your hair chromium would be a good idea, if you are serious about managing your bone structure.

- Focus on eating whole foods that are high in calcium. Now, there may be a lot of controversy over this, but I would personally avoid dairy (when was the last time you saw a cow eating cottage cheese, milk or ice cream? They eat hay, grass and alfalfa.) Instead, make sure you have greens everyday, sesame seeds and almonds (plant sources of calcium). At least have a source of organic almond butter.

- I would suggest a thyroid evaluation. See Chapter Seven on the Thyroid.

- Are you stressed? Most osteoporosis patients are to a point. If you have stress in your mind, your physical body can be impacted. As humans, the part of our brain that connects the emotional and physical halves does not necessarily differentiate between what is real and what is imaginary. Stress depletes the body of calcium. I caringly tell my patients to learn to say, "I can't say yes" when they are asked to be on another committee or commit to another project. They basically are saying "no" politely.

- What should you supplement with nutritionally? My suggestion would be the following:

    1. Have a mineral tissue analysis to determine levels of nutrients.

    2. Get a chemistry panel completed—especially request a serum, calcium and phosphorus reading. Have this completed while fasting. You want to make sure that your serum globulin level is at or above 2.7. Circulating globulin below 2.7 levels would suggest that

your body is not able to absorb protein, and you may not have adequate digestive acids to create an environment to absorb calcium.

3. Have a thyroid panel completed, including a TSH, T3 and T4. Go to Chapter Seven, the Thyroid chapter, for assessment.

4. Monitor your armpit temperature as discussed in the Thyroid Chapter. You would like to see it at or above 97.8°F.

5. We use a couple of products for long-term maintenance and structural support; Calcifood®, a source of veal bone, Biost® an item that promotes the utilization of Calcifood®, and Biodent®. I have had patients in their sixties reverse there bone destiny readings with supplementation and diet modification. Ligaplex II® is also beneficial; this formula is a great source of nutrients for long-term ligament integrity.

6. Monitor your bone density. Talk to your healthcare provider and have it done. Now there are screens that do it on the heel. You will want to use the same source or type. It may take up to two years to see reversal of your levels. Also, if your levels stay the same, that is success: you are not getting worse. The restoration of bone density also depends on how depleted you are, and on how many children you carried full term. Do not give up!

Take the results of the tests to an experienced Natural Healthcare provider, one familiar with assessing the findings. Generally, I find that I need to support the thyroid gland, and I commonly recommend a digestive aid. If you are in need of calcium, I recommend an easily absorbed, ionizable calcium lactate. In my practice, I also recommend a product called Calcifood® from Standard Process that has given excellent results. It is composed of wholesome ingredients including raw veal bone. This, in conjunction with an active enzyme called Biost® from the same company, has increased the bone density levels of my patients without tricking the osteoclasts.

NOTES_____

_____

_____

_____

_____

_____

_____

_____

_____

Proper Calcium Supplementation can prevent Poison Ivy

"I always knew that summer and poison ivy went hand in hand. What I didn't know was that they don't have to! In late May, when my daughter Christa was preparing to leave for her first summer camp counseling position, we stopped at Dr. Bob's to purchase some remedies to have on hand for when she would, inevitably, I thought, get poison ivy. I was surprised when Dr. Bob suggested something so she wouldn't get poison ivy in the first place! *I didn't know we had a choice in the matter! We left with a bottle of Calcium Lactate ® and L-lysine (Cataplex F® from Standard Process Labs can also be used to improve calcium absorption), and I'm happy to report that, after eight weeks on the job, Christa is the only counselor at her camp that has NOT gotten poison ivy! Instead, I got it. Weeding on our church property I encountered two small "suspicious vines," and not protected by the above named products, sure enough, I woke up with an eye that drooped like a basset hound. I was familiar with poison ivy manifesting as a rash, and while there was a little of that, droopy eyes were new to me. I figured the poison ivy would "run it's course" in a few days, like a cold. What a mistake! A few days later, I was in the emergency room of the hospital at four in the morning getting an IV with three meds. My ears were like Dumbo's, my head like a basketball and my big eyes were reduced to tiny slits. I felt like Fiona from* Shrek! *Later that morning, with multiple prescriptions to fill, I stopped by to ask Dr. Bob whether or not there was a natural alternative to Benadryl (an antihistamine that knocked me loopy!) and Prednisone (a cortisone-like drug.). Again, to my surprise, there was! Antronex® and Drenamin ® from Standard Process Labs were Dr. Bob's immediate recommendations, and the poison ivy cleared up.*

Thanks to Dr. Bob, I'll never again believe that poison ivy HAS to be part of my family's summer vacation, but even if it is, I now know a drugless alternative."

Patti Evans

10
Communication Between the Brain and Tissue Cells

The information that I would like to share with you in the next few pages is by far the single prevalent reason which separates what I do universally as a Natural Doctor versus a Western-trained allopathic physician. Healing comes from the inside out; cellular restoration does not come from the outside in. Putting pills and potions in or on the body only treats the symptoms. This is a very critical point worth repeating in order for you to understand what it takes for total, long-lasting restoration.

A successful surgery is actually an oxymoron. In other words, a successful surgery is one that never needed to have occurred. By that I mean, the patient should be instructed early enough in his/her life to engage in activities that promote life versus drain it. Empowering education of patients is vital if we want to help the next generations. The term doctor actually is translated from the Greek word, "Teacher."

This natural principle of healing from the inside out is dependent on your brain being able to communicate to each cell. Interruption of your body's ability to correspond would be very similar to you not receiving emails, phone calls, snail mail or text messages. Could you honestly live life to the fullest, as you know it now, without this communication? You would do best to incorporate whole food supplements to restore the nervous system versus seeking the healthcare provider who promotes symptomatic medical relief while denying the fact that the body functions with a brain cell to tissue cell connection. I have confronted innumerable healthcare providers who deny that the nervous system function is necessary for optimal health. Remember, once again, the Christopher Columbus story. I live it everyday.

It is a known fact and is described in anatomy books that the nervous system controls the functions of the body. The brain continues on as the spinal cord. The spinal cord is similar to the printer cable leaving your personal computer and connecting itself to your ancillary equipment like a printer or fax machine.

The nervous system is very sensitive and is actually protected by a bony conduit called the vertebral column. There are twenty-plus moveable parts to the conduit. The brain, your personal computer, is so important that it is protected by a bone case called your skull.

There are several nervous systems in the body that allow you to function without a conscious effort. Could you imagine if you needed to make a thinking effort to breathe, wink, pump your heart, move your bowels and release urine all simultaneously? I am not sure that you can even count your pulse and breathes for a minute. Go ahead and try it.

Visualize the front of your mind as the circuit panel that controls the power in your residence. If a switch is off to your refrigerator, how long would it take for the food to spoil so it could not be consumed without harming you? A day or two?

This actually happened to me a couple of years ago. A squirrel interrupted the flow of electricity from the transformer outside on the utility pole to the electric lines delivering power to the residences in my neighborhood. The electrical power was off to several thousands homes in the area. Fortunately for me, my neighbor is not on the same line, so I was able to connect to his source of electric power via a large electric cord and kept the vital appliances functioning. The food did not spoil because I responded very quickly. Your body will survive only milli-seconds when the main power is disconnected from the brain to the body.

I have a very significant point I want you to chew on. Do you see, smell or taste the electrons moving up and down the wires? No. But, knowing from experience, would you touch the end of an open cord or plug on an outlet without some kind of sensation? Of course not, you would get shocked. Well, here is the point. The brain is sending the same kind of living energy over the wires, or nerves, in your body. You cannot see it, feel it or touch it. The measuring of the power can be done by sophisticated equipment just like the power in electrical wiring can be assessed by a trained electrician.

Let's say the same event occurred and instead of reconnecting to another power source I called a family member who may have suggested that I go to the service station and purchase a bag of ice to keep the contents of the refrigerator cold. After several hours I would need to purchase another bag of ice. This would go on for hours. OK, by now the ice is melting and dripping on the carpet around the refrigerator and making a mess. This would be considered a bad or negative side effect. I may call another friend or relative and ask what would they do? It may be suggested to power up a generator or do what I did, find an alternate source of power. The body is not any different; if you do not have power, you will not work effectively.

"But, Dr. Bob, how does this process happen?" Let me ask you a question. Does gravity ever take a vacation? The answer is NO. So what occurs is that gravity is continuously and relentlessly compressing the very sensitive nerves that are nestled between two vertebrae. Compound that with the facts that you may have poor sleep and postural habits that cause spinal compromise, you bend and twist at work and play, you more than likely have been in several traumatic accidents, and you may have started life with a strenuous birth process like an unnatural surgical cesarean section, all of which can create an environment for spinal and communication network breakdown.

The compression itself can impair the flow of electrical current from the brain to the organ that is waiting for a message. If this happens, over time the organ or organs will not know exactly what to do, and as they become more disconnected from their power source, they start to malfunction. I have seen this phenomenon occur hundreds of thousands of times in my career. You, yes you, may be suffering needlessly right now because no one ever told you that you should be checked for mis-alignment in your spine that is choking the nerves.

The reason I am also so focused on what a person eats is because what you eat affects the integrity of the spinal structure. Water increases the size of the disc height between the vertebrae. Smoking and sugar depletes the mineral structure in those same discs causing them to compress prematurely. We are talking about a complete orchestra that is interdependent on each member for the unit to work in a symphonic melody.

I need to relate to you a condition that occurs in females that is a prime example of what I am talking about and have successfully helped restore on innumerable occasions. By now, you should have learned that the ovaries need to be fueled with minerals, protein, vitamins, oils and especially iodine to operate at peak performance. You should also realize that the ovaries create hormones, especially progesterone to balance estrogen. I have had patients, and I am sure this has happened to many of you, who have a post-menstrual headache one month and the next month do not have a post-menstrual headache. Right, so here is what is going on.

The patient can be living with a subluxation in the lower part of the spine and pelvic-sacral area that is interrupting the performance of the ovary by impeding the transfer of communication from the brain. The subluxation impairment needs only to be on one side of the body and the month when it is that ovary's turn to work, it is not capable of doing so. How do I know this? Because many women suffer with a German-named condition called Mittlesmerz. Mittlesmerz is a term used to denote a painful ovary. When the ovary is in pain, do you think it is working at its best? Hardly. By the way, you don't have to feel pain to know if the ovary is or is not functioning properly. Chasing pain does not answer all the questions, and you really should not cover up pain with a medication.

I have on many occasions adjusted the lower spine with a specific spinal correction, and over time, the patient returns and tells me that not only did the ovarian pain stop, but in that same month there was no headache and, in fact, she is headache free. Was it a placebo effect? I know that is what well-meaning allopathic physicians would say, but I can tell you this: I have many very well-educated, female patients that would be insulted if you even suggested that it was a placebo. Most of these same patients have repeatedly told their physicians about their ovarian pain, and the physician looked at the patient with a glaring stare, communicating with body language that said the physician really couldn't help them. I have helped a lot of women labeled as hypochondriacs, who were in fact living with subluxation which was interfering with the body's e-mail system. Do you understand what I am saying? This may be YOU!! For your WHOLE LIFE!!

What happened was simple to say the least. The ovary was finally able to receive the information from which it had been disconnected. I have come to the conclusion, after seeing this so many times and for many different conditions, that the organs literally go into a state of self-imposed hibernation and get by with what little information they can get in order to survive. Over time, if this is not corrected or relieved, the body starts to break down, and you have a state of poor function. Now, not to scare you, this can take years. The good news is that, in many cases, if we motivate the patient to make appropriate lifestyle modifications, feed the body correctly, get checked for proper spinal alignment and reduce subluxation patterns, the body will improve itself to the best it is capable of doing. I have witnessed total and full recovery of some of the most intense diagnosed conditions with the sequence I just wrote. I am excited to help YOU!!

I want to share with you another analogy. I see this occur in nature and I believe it will help those of you who may not have body signals of poor ovary function. Have you ever seen a branch on a tree that has little barnacle growing on it? If you were to go up close and investigate the tree and branch you will probably see the rest of the tree is growing and flourishing, but for whatever reason this branch may seem dry and brittle. Upon further study you may actually see a small break in the bark itself.

The branch has been disconnected from its source. The barnacles are nature's way of decomposing the unnecessary burden to the tree. Over time the branch may fall in a wind or ice storm. Organs that are not functioning in the body are similar to the branch. When the organ becomes a burden to the body, you will start to experience poor body function. The organ is breaking down or decomposing slowly. Sometimes the symptoms you may be suffering with may not even be related to the organ itself but to a detoxifying organ like the liver, colon or kidneys trying to process the debris.

You may, and this happens more often than not, see your family healthcare provider who assesses poor function. You may then be referred to a specialist who isolates the primary organ not operating as efficiently as needed for the body as a whole. It may then be determined that in order for you to survive, this malfunctioning tissue needs to be removed. So, you go through with the surgery and feel great for a season. Then, what happens when your body has determined that all the parts are not there anymore? You start having other breakdown phenomenon and the cycle continues.

The real challenge is how to assist you if an organ is removed. Well, first we need to make sure that we have all the remaining organs receiving the vital information from the brain so they are able to contribute most efficiently in order to support the system. It is not possible to restore the body to its pre-surgical status.

Here is some solid structural information for your spine, nervous system and posture to operate optimally. Your posture is the window to your spine. If your spine is not in proper alignment — with aligned frontal or front to side position – your posture is not optimal. When your posture is compromised, your nervous system is not going to function as well. I have included a set of exercise maneuvers that you need to complete on a daily basis. Remember gravity does not take a day off. A healthy spine is a healthy you.

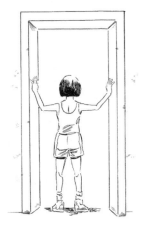

I advise my patients to perform these maneuvers on a regular basis:

The Door Jam Push-Up is a simple maneuver designed to pull the shoulders back. A forward head position is not a healthy posture alignment. Stand in a door jam (it can be imaginary). Raise your hands to shoulder height or above, place the palms on the door jam and lean your body into the doorway. Hold this five seconds. Do three sets of 15 daily.

The ball exercise is awesome. You may want to find an accountability partner to do these with. Your goal is to have your head resting with your ears right about to the center of your shoulder tip.

Also, your tummy needs to be pulled backward. I would encourage you to get on all fours, whether in bed or on the floor, and push your back up towards the ceiling; this is fondly called the "cat stretch." Regular anti-gravity exercising will go a long way to managing your hormone issues.

You are going to want to have your spinal structure assessed by a passionate, skilled spinal specialist. When I am asked for an out-of-town referral, I encourage individuals to ask around. Go to a health-food store, talk to a personal fitness trainer, yoga instructor or someone who understands how structure works. I would personally seek the hands of a subluxation-based chiropractor that has studied and is knowledgeable in diet and nutrition.

You need to take some action and it is OK to go in and interview the doctor. This is your body you are talking about. Another important point for you to remember is that it took time for you to get this way and it will take time for the body to repair itself. The doctor does not do the healing — your body does. His job description is to help remove the interference; your job is to do what you can to manage function. Drink water; eat whole foods, exercise and rest.

DO YOU HAVE ANY OF THESE SYMPTOMS?

- Look at yourself in the mirror. Is your posture perpendicular to the floor?
- Can you bend over and touch your toes without pain?
- Close your eyes and turn your head left and right. Do you hear grinding?

♦ Obtain two scales. Stand on them both at the same time. Do you weigh more on one side? If you are not balanced you may have a spinal structural weakness.

If any of the above findings are positive or you are not balanced, you would do best to locate a skilled chiropractor who works with his/her hands and takes postural spinal films.

NOTES_____

_____

_____

_____

_____

_____

_____

_____

PART II

LEARN HOW TO WAKE UP THE DETECTIVE INSIDE OF YOU

11
Common Female Conditions That Are Challenging

You may be plagued with a variety of other hormonal-based conditions that I have not yet focused on. Let me explain to you why I have not discussed all the possibilities. I have come to the conclusion that most of the challenges women suffer with are precipitated by the same factors, i.e., poor diet choices, toxic build up and sabotaged communication between the brain cells and the tissue cells. I do not want you to think I am not concerned about endometriosis, enlarged uteruses, dysplasia, breast and/or ovarian cysts. I am. Truthfully, I would not tell you anything different in the way of cause and treatment. You need to focus on what you are putting in and on your body. You must evaluate what you are doing to yourself.

Let me give you an interesting example of what I am talking about. I have the opportunity to treat many generations of patients. I have one such family where I have been privileged to help a grandmother, her daughter, granddaughter and great granddaughter. They are awesome and understand the role of natural choice in the overall health pattern. The daughter was in the hospital for several days with idiopathic pain (unknown cause of chest pain). She had seen my Natural Health program on TV and said to herself, "I need to see Dr. Bob." She checked herself out of the hospital and came into the office. I completed my normal intake procedure and determined that through trauma and injury she had rotated or misaligned a rib. I made a specific, corrective maneuver and immediately her gnawing pain diminished. Upon further counseling, I explained to her that the food she was eating (sweet fruits and potatoes) may have created a reflex that threw off the messages from her viscera (organs) to her spine. This is a very common complaint that responds well to natural drugless treatment. Medicine does not totally understand this cause and effect scenario. They think "outside in."

She was so excited about what we were able to do for her that she asked me to assess her sixteen-year-old daughter who was a model. The very attractive young woman came into my office with very typical issues for a teen: acne, headaches and menstrual pain. Mom was most concerned because she had been told she had a cyst on her breast and she needed to have a biopsy. The young lady was told to stop drinking and consuming items with caffeine; a normal protocol suggestion to anyone with cysts on their breast. I was very inquisitive and started asking more questions such as what types of lotions and/or creams she put on her body? She was applying a common "baby gel" so her skin would be smooth and vibrant. I have access to a microscope, so we examined the integrity of her blood under a "live state." Much to her surprise, but not uncommon in my experience, she had what appeared as little "fat globules" in her specimen. I believe, that what was going on with her was, that her skin and lymphatic system were absorbing the material causing the body to be overwhelmed and unable to process the foreign substance (sodium lauryl sulfate). The body deposited it in the breast tissue, a common reservoir for women in a toxic state (breast cysts). She stopped using the product and has not had a problem since. I strongly advise you to review the American Cancer Society's list of items that are cancerous and eliminate them from your cosmetics and lotions. Many common ingredients in lotions are actually quite toxic.

Any item that alters the normal physiology of female hormones has the potential to create an abnormal cell response. Birth control pills are dispensed today to teenagers for a variety of body signals including acne, depression and/or irregular and painful menses. I have seen many young teens on birth control pills who were chronically ill. They present with various menstrual challenges including severe menses headaches. My experience suggests that women at any age who have been taking any type of synthetic female hormone, for whatever reason, have the potential to develop abnormal side effects. The aberrant effects are the body's response and attempt to normalize some type of equilibrium in the system. The medical community's answer to emotional challenges today seems to be an antidepressant and/or birth control pill. Focus on putting the right fuel into the system would be a more appropriate answer.

A lifestyle of soda and French fries, with a focus on low fat, high carbohydrate convenience and snack foods is hardly fueling the body correctly. If you are a mom reading this, it is critical for you to relay this information to your daughter. In what seems like a very short time period, she could be facing ablation, hysterectomy, biopsies on breast tissue and ovary cyst removal, because of the consequences of toxic food choices. Conventional medicine continues to focus on and create the mindset that nearly all health issues today are the result of some renegade genes from inherited DNA. I treat families where one family member is attentive to their eating and exercise habits and does not have distress. They ask me questions on how a sibling in another location is facing radical hormonal and/or surgical intervention. The difference is lifestyle choices.

I have treated all of the previously mentioned conditions the same way. Do an assessment on all the glands and functions I have discussed thus far in the book, and treat them accordingly. I commonly and consistently find estrogen saturation and toxic build up. I have had women come into the office with a history of large fibroids on their uterus combined with elevated estrogen levels. After making a decision to change everything about their life, the fibroid stopped growing and, in fact, diminished over time.

I have a patient who is an RN, a personal fitness trainer and once worked for an Obstetrician/Gynecologist. She came to my office with multiple cysts on her ovaries that have since been reduced by adding more protein to her diet. This same patient had fat phobia and never ate the yolk in her egg. She also was literally addicted to soy lattes. Needless to say, she was reading all the latest information in magazines focused on women's health. She was doing everything right! WRONG!

She was headed for disaster. She was addicted to sugar and had chronic left neck and shoulder blade pain, and she suffered with a chronic sore throat. She was a mess, like some of you reading this book. Well, where would you start? I started by suggesting she take flax oil, one tablespoon per one hundred pounds of body weight, drink water from a pure source and stop the soy lattés! Most soy milks used at coffee houses have sugar in them. I strongly encouraged her to eat more protein. She listened to everything I said and guess what happened? All of her body signals improved. It took a little over twelve months, but it happened. She now has a regular menstrual cycle, her throat is better, and the craving for sweets is also gone. This same scenario can and does happen to people just like you.

"OK, but Dr. Bob, I have a mom and aunts that have suffered with cysts and tumors the size of grapefruits on their uteruses and ovaries, and I do not want cysts and tumors." I understand your concern. You need to change the recipe box. Stop eating and drinking what they eat and drink and start the proactive recommendations I have suggested. Most of all, stop eating partially-hydrogenated or trans fat, or your body will incorporate those fats into cell membranes and you will have mutation of cells. This is very serious — I am sure you understand that.

So, regardless of whatever condition you may be suffering with, what you have done to this point in your life must change. If you do not change, whatever the named condition is, it will continue to proliferate and interrupt your life.

Your goal is to clean up your habits, eat whole food, drink water from a pure source and do not consume any extra toxins. That may mean you will want to stop drinking alcohol. Having two drinks a day can increase your statistical chances of having breast cancer by twenty-five percent. You must realize that I am describing natural principles; you cannot get a "hall pass" or skip school that day and get away with it. Your body, when abused and tested long enough, will start to break down.

Let me put it to you this way. Whatever condition you suffer, and whatever name has been placed on it, it will respond if you make the changes I have suggested. Now, unfortunately, you may be at a point where your body has been beaten up so badly that it cannot turn itself around. Do not give up! I have seen the most serious conditions respond, if you do everything I have mentioned. I have had patients who came into my office with only months to live but have gone on to live five years or more, without medication and chemotherapy. I am currently seeing an elderly female who came into my office thirty years ago with cancer. She specifically told me she was diagnosed with cancer and was concerned about her health. That was thirty years ago. She recently told me, and I have heard this more than once, that the biggest challenge she has had is finding new friends, because hers have passed on.

I want you to have an increased quality of life. So, understand this, your body will do what it needs to do. Follow the steps to optimal health.

JUST TELL ME WHAT TO DO

- The key, regardless of your diagnosis, is not to get carried away and start taking a lot of different medicines or best-friend-suggested synthetic supplements and doing "outside in" treatment.

- Review the Estrogen, Liver and Cleansing Chapters (Two, Six and Seventeen). Your goal is to cleanse the system.

- You may want to start with a saliva assessment of your estrogen and progesterone levels. If the estrogen is high and progesterone is low, your focus needs to be to elevate the progesterone and lower the estrogen, which is the most common scenario I see with nearly all common female health issues. The liver needs to be supported. You will want to make sure you are taking adequate whole food B vitamins and NO SUGAR!

- If you choose to pursue another assessment to locate the cause of your challenge, you may want to start with the Thyroid panel. That will give you an idea of your thyroid function and the amount of iodine in your body. If you're T3 and T4 are low, you need to make sure you are taking twelve milligrams of iodine a day. I use Prolamine Iodine® from Standard Process Labs. Your ovaries need the iodine to make progesterone to counter balance the extra estrogen.

- Take your morning armpit temperature when you do the thyroid panel and monitor the degrees as a gauge of your progress. Do the same with your blood pressure, sitting to standing. You can monitor your progress by assessing these simple tests as you follow your protocols.

- Start taking one tablespoon per one hundred pounds of body weight of organic flax oil a day. I use the High Lignan Omega Flow product from Omega Nutrition.

- Avoid all processed food and drinks; drink water from a pure source.

- Start exercising regularly. This means work something into your daily schedule.

- Be assessed by a spinal subluxation, nutritionally-based chiropractor. Contact Standard Process Labs to find one in your area, if you do not already have a family chiropractor.

- Take the appropriate supplements that are recommended from your testing results. Go to the Supplement Chapter, Eighteen, and treat accordingly. You will want to be monitored by your natural healthcare provider.

- I would suggest you eliminate any synthetic, chemical female hormones, including birth control pills. Also, once your adrenal function is up to par, I would eliminate progesterone creams. Your body should be well on its way to making its own. Review the symptoms of excesses and deficiencies in Chapter Two on Estrogen and Chapter Three on Progesterone.

NOTES_____

_____

_____

_____

_____

_____

_____

_____

12
What Causes Hot Flashes?

I would like to discuss hot flashes, which are one of the primary reasons why women will go to their healthcare provider for an opinion. Assistance for hot flashes and night sweats can be provided by the use of natural protocols. If you suffer from either hot flashes or night sweats, you're not alone. In fact, 85 percent of women in the U.S. experience some form of hot flashes during pre, peri and post menopause and in the year or two following menopause. I have new patients in their late seventies who come into the office still having hot flashes, and also many who have never had them. When you compare the lifestyles of the various individuals, with or without hot flashes, you can see how diet and emotional states are a part of the dilemma.

Fifty percent of women will experience hot flashes for years after menopause when they have not received care or are not at optimal health. We treat and support their adrenal glands, thyroid and overall whole body function without a patch or cream. We do it internally with your own natural body chemistry restoration; all without soy.

Whether you get them all the time or just once in a while, hot flashes can be extremely disruptive to your life. They're not only embarrassing and distracting, but can sometimes even be scary.

For many, the worst aspect of hot flashes is the sense of powerlessness over your own body.

It's true that during peri-menopause, menopause and while weaning off hormone replacement therapy (HRT), your body is going through a major hormonal transition. The good news is that you can use this time to get in touch with your body and your health and in the process you can learn to control or eliminate your hot flashes naturally and without drugs. The body's response to stressful situations and environments is a part of the scenario. How you feed your body and the state of your overall health determines the reaction. I have had patients in my office have a hot flash when they were confronted with a simple question or statement that was not significant, but to them it was a major obstacle. I am always amazed at how there are so many females that are not aware of how their body reacts to situations and food. They haven't been taught to read how their own system works.

I recently had a thirty-nine-year-old female MD start care. She had been on the "medical merry-go-round" without any type of success or satisfaction for her trigger fingers (when a small nodule develops in the tendons of the palm of your hand and fingers), the bronzing on the sides of her cheeks (liver and adrenal gland stress), hip pain, headaches and loss of libido. She was at her wits' end when a personal fitness trainer and a massage therapist suggested she receive natural care. I discussed with her exactly what I am telling you in this book, and within two weeks, her hip pain was gone, she had no more wrist and hand pain, her headaches were history and the breast tenderness she lived with for years during the latter part of her menstrual cycle was gone. Needless to say, she was very happy. It does not make any difference who you are; physiology or cell function is cell function, MD, DC, DO, ND, PhD or someone just like you.

HOW DO I KNOW IT'S A HOT FLASH?

The symptoms associated with hot flashes vary from woman to woman. Some women feel hot all the time, while others experience flashes. Here are some physical and psychological symptoms associated with hot flashes and night sweats:

- ☐ An intense feeling of heat in the face and upper body
- ☐ Increased heart rate
- ☐ Dizziness
- ☐ Nausea
- ☐ Headache
- ☐ Perspiration
- ☐ Weakness
- ☐ Feeling suffocated
- ☐ Anxiety
- ☐ Flushed appearance or blotchy skin
- ☐ Chills as the hot flash subsides

WHAT CAUSES HOT FLASHES?

The long-held belief that hot flashes are caused by too little estrogen is not totally agreed upon. There are multiple factors leading to hot flashes, and the truth is that during natural menopause, estrogen levels don't fall until later in the transition. Body signals that include hot flashes are most likely the result of a shift in the balance between estrogen and progesterone; and it is progesterone that is usually low, not estrogen. You can assess yourself by having a saliva assessment of your progesterone and estrogen levels. Record your hot flash activity during the month while you are measuring your levels. There are no consistent factors that are common in women with the rise and fall of their temperature.

You may be surprised that there will be more hot flash body signals when your adrenal glands are stressed. The adrenal glands and ovaries are your main sources of progesterone. This is one of the reasons I have consistently seen hot flashes in my patients with lumbar subluxation (See Chapter Ten on Communication). You can understand why many patients will have relief of their hot flashes with spinal correction, which corrects the communication to the ovaries, and changing their diet. It is the secret weapon and reason why so many chiropractors see improvement with this common condition. The ovaries can once again produce the progesterone needed. Actually, the body will create the correct balance of either estrogen or progesterone, whichever needs to be innately corrected. You are waking up the pharmacist in you. Unfortunately, patients are not properly instructed nor do they follow through with dietary changes to minimize stress on the endocrine or hormone system. You can take up to twelve milligrams of iodine daily to feed the ovaries. I would avoid soy since it is an anti-thyroid food as well as sugar, which is an anti-adrenal food. You want all the organs operating at their best. Feed the body right!

An interesting finding that I see in my female patients with hot flashes, is that they have tenderness of the cartilage along the breast bone. I often see this body signal in low thyroid function. It is called Tietze syndrome. You would do best to follow the protocol in the Chapter Seven: Fuel theThyroid to Keep the Body Going, to support your thyroid and ovaries.

Whether you are suffering from hot flashes due to the natural fluctuation of your hormones during peri-menopause and menopause or because of rapidly weaning off HRT, the physiology is very similar. A menopausal hot flash is essentially caused by a mix-up of signals between the brain and the body. As your hormones naturally shift during peri-menopause and menopause, some women's brains receive confused messages from their bodies and hot flashes result. The brain, in particular, is affected by fluctuations in estrogen that occur against a backdrop of relatively low levels of progesterone. During moments of extreme estrogen flux, the temperature-regulatory part of the hypothalamus (the CEO of your body, See Chapter One on hormones) misinterprets the message as a signal for elevated core body heat. It responds by sending "release heat" messages to the peripheral body.

To release this heat, the body reacts within seconds by increasing its heart rate and dilating vessels to circulate more blood, as well as opening sweat glands. For some women, waves of anxiety wash over them, while others might feel heart palpitations. When it's all over, the uncomfortable sensations and panic may have passed, but you're left in a puddle of sweat.

The sudden impulse to dispel the body of heat is a built-in mechanism to protect us from overheating in intensely warm situations, as in the throes of exercise, stress or infection. But when a hot flash overtakes us, we are not truly over heating; the brain just thinks we are. This confusion between body and brain can be mighty uncomfortable and can increase skin temperature by several degrees.

The rash of flushing events and hormonal storms generally subside a couple of years into menopause. Some women, however, will continue to experience them well into their menopausal years. And for women trying to taper off HRT after menopause, hot flashes can return as a result of hormone withdrawal and subsequent fluctuation of estrogen.

The specific triggers for hot flashes and night sweats are as colorful and varied as women are themselves, which is why there is no one-size-fits-all solution.

WHY ONLY SOME WOMEN SUFFER HOT FLASHES

Just as triggers vary, so do hot flashes in general. In fact, some of our mothers and grandmothers never experienced hot flashes or night sweats at all. Even today, many women in the world make a far calmer and cooler menopausal transition than those in the United States.

The reasons underlying these cultural differences are several-fold. The absence of hot flashes may be the result of a less erratic course of hormonal fluctuation during this stage of life, different diets and exercise patterns or because the brain simply doesn't get its messages mixed up. A transition free of hot flashes may also be a result of better coping mechanisms for stress or having solid measures of support already set in place for the elevated demands placed on the body during this time of change.

Although some women have an easier time than others, on the whole, it seems as though today's menopausal women are suffering more from hot flashes than in the past. This is likely due to our changing world, stressful lifestyles (adrenal gland stress), and how we support our systems nutritionally and emotionally. Women in midlife today are pulled in many directions: between caring for older and younger generations, full-time jobs, house-hold demands, marital challenges and financial concerns; our plates are full of responsibilities. I consistently see adrenal stress simultaneously with individuals with hot flashes. The adrenal glands are your back-up source of progesterone, and estrogen needs to be functioning optimally, along with the thyroid, to make it through the menopause journey without hot flashes.

At the same time, the quality of our food supply and eating patterns are not what they once were. Diets high in refined carbohydrates and processed foods result in less resilience to otherwise normal hormonal changes in the menopausal years. Partially hydrogenated or trans fat interferes with and sabotages the formation of long chain fats and fat metabolism, all of which are needed for hormone function. These oils have been commonly added to our foods the last thirty or forty years or so. Amish women do not consume trans fat and do not have the same issues with hot flashes like their English counterparts.

But the good news is, no matter what your health foundation or how severe your hot flashes and night sweats, your body has an amazing ability to heal when you learn to listen to its messages and take steps to provide it support.

HOT FLASH AND/OR NIGHT SWEAT TRIGGERS

It's helpful to identify underlying causes or triggers of hot flashes. Try tracking your hot flashes in a diary or journal. Are there certain times of the day when you are more prone to having a hot flash or do your night flashes wake you at a particular time of the night? Are there foods that seem to set you off on a heat wave? Here are some of the triggers, including foods to avoid, for hot flashes:

- Sugar foods, sweet fruits that act like sugar in the system and simple carbohydrates (bananas, raisins and grapes)
- Caffeine, nicotine and stimulants in general
- Alcohol (including wine)
- Spicy foods and hot (temperature) drinks or foods
- Hot places, such as saunas, hot tubs, showers and overly warm bedrooms
- Anxiety or stressful events or people (Adrenal Stress)
- Exercise or any type of activity that heats the body up without allowing adequate cool-down time

While some women see a clear correlation between their hot flashes and triggers, others find it more difficult to make these connections. Once you track your hot flashes for a week or two you're very likely to spot patterns in how, when, where and why you get them most. From that point, a plan to address the triggers will be able to be developed.

HELP FOR HOT FLASHES

Antidepressant use, a solution conventional medicine is turning to for hot flash relief, is not an approach ever used at our office. It does not get to the cause of the problem. Often, depression is a result of inadequate nutrients needed for thyroid function; L-tyrosine, an amino acid protein building block, helps to diminish the symptoms of depression.

I have been prescribing natural solutions that effectively address the underlying causes of hot flashes and have provided results for over 30 years. My approach to resolving hot flashes includes:

- Dietary and nutritional support
- Lifestyle modifications
- Gentle, natural endocrine support with whole food supplements
- Improving spinal function and reducing subluxation

Time and again we find that the majority of women experience rapid and marked reduction in their hot flashes and other hormonal symptoms by feeding the body right and cleaning out the liver.

DIET AND NUTRITIONAL SUPPORT

Experience has shown us that women get amazing results by giving their bodies the nutrition they need. Eating a balanced diet of protein, healthy organic (not man-made synthetic) fats (flax and or black currant seed oil), complex carbohydrates (especially vegetables), and select fruits (as I mentioned earlier, I do not encourage sweet fruits such as bananas, raisins, grapes, pineapple and any dried fruit) and vegetables provides your body and brain with the building materials it needs to function and keeps signals from getting crossed. An easy way to add protein to your diet and help hormonal fluctuations is by adding small portions of protein throughout the day. Almond butter, organic deli meats, hard boiled eggs and egg white protein with almond, rice or oat milk are great additions. This is important: I do not encourage soy. Note: A source of information on soy and its impact on health can be found at the Soy Online Service (Google), and in particular, its page on phyto-estrogenic effects of soy, and impact on the thyroid, a key player in the endocrine hormonal system. Also a great book, *Why Am I always Tired?* By Anne Louise Gittleman Ph.D., will help you understand the reason soy can be an issue.

There are too many conflicting results using soy. Patients continually obtain great improvement without being on it, and even better when they get off it. Remember, a balanced diet provides building materials which contribute to your hormones and neurotransmitters, both of which affect hot flashes and your overall sense of well being.

I suggest using a whole food multiple supplement such as Catalyn® from Standard Process Labs. I have also seen hot flashes disappear by adding a quality sourced organic flax oil. I suggest the flax oil with high lignans from Omega Nutrition; one tablespoon per one hundred pounds. These two items alone will help bridge any gap in a basic nutrition program and ensure the adequate supply of nutrients your body needs for neuro-transmitter and hormonal balance. Your body needs these items when creating long chain fatty acids in the fat metabolism pathway.

Stress is finally being recognized by conventional medicine as a significant factor in the cause of hot flashes. In my evaluation of women with hot flashes, their histories and consultations have revealed a direct correlation between anxiety and the severity and frequency of their hot flashes.

Deep paced breathing and relaxation exercises performed throughout the day significantly decrease the frequency and severity of flushing symptoms; further supporting the precept of stress as a major trigger. I have so many female patients who, not only have a full-time occupation creating income for the home, but they also juggle caring for their children, aging parents, spouses and community activities. They are super moms, existing in a world that is pulling at them from all directions. The body can only take so much before it yells for help. Could that be the time hot flashes start?

If you know that relaxing is what you need to calm your hot flashes, you might try a behavioral therapy of quiet time and focus on events and moments that are calming. Many times our health depends heavily on our emotional state. Just as certain foods and drugs can be toxic to your system, <u>stress and negative emotions can also be toxic</u>.

Anger is an emotion that mind-body practitioners relate to problems with the liver, and in turn, is often implicated in hot flashes. Learn to identify and navigate negative emotions accordingly and find ways to give yourself more time for relaxation and re-energizing. There is a great book that goes into detail on how to navigate your emotions. It was a part of my curriculum for my NHD degree, *The Relaxation and Stress Reduction Workbook,* by Martha Davis Ph.D., Elizabeth Robbins Eshelman, MSW, and Mathew M. Kay, Ph.D.

There is also little doubt that exercise is one of the best things you can do to calm your body and mind. Experience has shown that hot flashes are yet another health concern that exercise can help with, principally by reducing anxiety. Menopausal patients who participated in exercise classes, at the office with my trainer, noticed the effect of their exercises on their personal, overall menopause symptoms. The exercises proved to reduce hot flashes. While those with menopausal symptoms and did not exercise, showed an increase in hot flashes.

When it comes to exercise, however, I recommend that you time your activity so the exercises do you the most good. You may want to do your exercises in the morning or midday, following natural cortisol levels in the body. By exercising consistently at night, you are not allowing your adrenal glands to rest like they should. It is also better to avoid dashing off to undertake activities that are stressful or involve a high level of activity directly following your workouts. The stress of fitting exercise into your life can be counter-productive so, make sure it is timed right, and you are not overtaxing your day planner or yourself.

Make a commitment to reducing stress, whatever form it takes in your life, even if you have to chip away at it one degree at a time. Whether that means setting better boundaries at work, home or within your community, learn to value your own well-being enough to say "No."

JUST TELL ME WHAT TO DO

- I would suggest starting with your axillary (armpit) temperature as discussed in Chapter Seven on the thyroids. Use that as a gauge to see how your core temperature is doing. If it is less than 97.8°F, you may want to pursue TSH, T3 and T4 testing. Review the Thyroid Chapter to see how.

- Is your breast bone tender; Tiezte syndrome? This is commonly seen in my office with women who have hot flashes. Avoid soda; it is throwing off your calcium metabolism which can create sternum (breast bone) chest area rib pain.

- Have your blood pressure taken while lying down or sitting; then have it done in the standing position. If it drops, I would suggest you may want to review Chapter Eight on the adrenal glands and support accordingly.

- Avoid sugar, pastries and other refined foods.

- Find an exercise that you like, at an appropriate time, and be consistent.

- Take one tablespoon of flax oil per one hundred pounds of body weight, avoid trans fat and other fake fats.

- I would avoid soy products for a month if you have severe hot flashes. Especially avoid coffee with soy milk.

- Add deep breathing exercises to your life.

- Find a quiet place and relax regularly.

- Organize your day and incorporate your entire family in the household chores to reduce your stress levels.

- If you are craving salt, use Celtic Sea Salt®. You can use it liberally. Your body is seeking minerals as fast as you are burning them in your stressful life. Minerals are essential to make fat for hormones.

- Follow these steps. You are healing your body from the inside out. Give it time. Please take time to rest.

NOTES_____

_____

_____

_____

_____

_____

_____

Patient Testimony:

"The hormonal issues that I had before making lifestyle changes were mainly hot flashes and depression. I was taking three kinds of depression medications over the years. I was also taking Ibuprofen and Excedrin for headaches. Following Dr. Bob's advice, I cut out sugar altogether, and I also cut back on coffee and tea (I'm still working on these). It has been difficult cutting back on coffee, tea and chocolate. I also have a problem with salt. I am cutting back, but it's really a struggle. I also eat more vegetables.

The only hormonal issue I currently have is a periodic episode of "night sweats" (if I deviate from my diet). Everything else has gone away. I am completely off the depression medicine, and I hardly have any headaches. If I do, they are minor. I seem to have lots more energy, and I'm not as sick with colds or flu. I always feel good after my adjustments. I feel younger, happier and enjoy doing things. My life is definitely better!" **Janet Crumley**

Information and documents in part cited from: Marcy Holmes, NP, Certified Menopause Clinician found at:
http://www.womentowomen.com/menopause/hotflashesnights weats.asp

13

Learning From the Amish

I want to share some insightful information with you. I have a colleague that has been treating Amish families for years. He also treats "the English," the name the Amish affectionately call us typical Americans. He may assess four or five hundred Amish patients every week. I have spent time with him at one of the farms where he treats his patients. I had an opportunity to walk through their homes, barns and outside areas and see how they live day-to-day and what they eat. What a wonderful experience. It was like going back over one hundred years, before electricity was in every remote area in the world. I posed several questions to him about the patients he treated before I decided to pass on this information to you.

Have you ever been to an Amish farm? Do you think they have stress? Have you ever seen a buggy traffic jam? Would you get up everyday and milk cows? Would you miss an electric dryer? Would you want to eat lima beans, corn or squash for a week straight?

Now, I am not saying that the Amish do not eat a variety of food or have time off. I want to make the point that they live today like we did as a society fifty or sixty years ago when Americans had limited conveniences. Can you imagine not having the conveniences of your life? Would you want to do your daily activities without electricity?

Being an Amish person in America without all the conveniences versus being someone with electricity is tougher than you might think. They will participate in our lifestyle to a degree, but they do not own our conveniences. For instance, the Amish will pay for drivers to take them where they need to go.

One critical item that really separates what they eat versus what we eat is the fact that they do not eat trans fat. The food they eat is food they prepare. They grow their own produce which has not been processed and still has the original components in it.

The fact that they only eat food grown on farms in their own area is quite significant. I have read several articles over time which suggested that you should eat food within a three hundred and fifty mile range of where you live. I am of the observation that the consumers in America today eat food from distant lands and climates which are often picked prior to full ripening and then sprayed with various gases to create coloration that would represent and create taste appeal. These altered foods are not quite physiologically right and may create distress to the system, especially pain syndromes and digestive distress.

Let's say you live in a southern, warm climate. It is best to focus on foods that are cooling such as fruits and water based light vegetables versus dense starch items. Foods that cool should be consumed in the summer and warm climates, and not in the winter time. You would want to focus on roots and squashes grown in the North versus a lot of southern climate food if you live in a cold region. I know this may seem new to you. However, I have seen a lot of chronic pain syndromes go away just by having my northern based, cold climate patients avoid citrus during the winter. The Amish do not have to be concerned about that because they eat their own food which is grown locally. Your goal is to create a lifestyle that has the least amount of stress to the system.

I primarily eat food that is organic, and I can tell you there is a taste difference between conventionally grown items and organic produced foods. Organic radishes have a crunch and a sensation that creates an electrifying zing in your tongue. You can taste the unique flavor in beans versus the bland, tasteless consistency of beans that have been commercially grown in dead, devitalized soil, sprayed to keep the bugs off and then canned. Do you know what the Amish use as fertilizer? They use the manure from their animals, not toxic chemicals that have the potential to cause the list of issues I have discussed thus far.

The Amish preserve their own food by home canning, and they keep it in cool cellars below or next to their homes. They also dig large pits in the ground to store the vegetables through the winter, like the farmers in America did only a generation ago. They live off the land and enjoy the fruits of their labor knowing well what they are eating.

Have you ever looked at the list of ingredients on the label of a food container? Can you pronounce all the names? The best food to eat, according to one of my patients, is food with no label on it. Yes, you read it right. When was the last time you saw a label on cauliflower, broccoli or cucumbers.

Researchers would have you thinking that the stress of modern daily living is the reason you are having your hot flashes, emotional and hormonal distress. The Amish have stress in their way of living, but they do not know any different. Their overall health is not what you think it would be. They get sick, have colds and chronic infections just like we do. However, they do not appear to have the same exhausted hormonal issues that are plaguing Western women: osteoporosis, hot flashes and hysterectomies.

Posturally, you do not see senior Amish women walking around all hunched over. They have a strong structure that serves them well into their senior years. The older Amish folks live with their children and grandchildren. So, there is a continuation of family purpose and continuity. We have many blended families today, and that, along with divorce, makes it challenging for the family network to give the support needed. The additional burden created by a challenged family life results in adrenal gland stress and a drain on the hormonal system.

According to my colleague's observations, the Amish do not have osteoporosis near to the degree of the English; 15 percent of the Amish have bony changes demonstrated on x-ray compared to 85 percent for the English in his East Coast practice. I asked him why he thought this was the case. He promptly said "the Amish work hard everyday. They work in the field, in the barn and in the home. They are used to being labor intensive. They eat whole food that they make themselves from scratch." Not a normal way of doing it in our "English" society today. It is like the coral story. They are active from the beginning of their lives and continue until they pass on.

Amish children have a lot of responsibility for the existence and survival of the family unit, unlike their English counterparts. They also enjoy playing outside and have fun in the sun, using their imaginations and creativity.

An interesting side point that I have learned from my patients, who have been involved in behavioral and brain health issues, is regarding the lack of exercise and activities of the hand. I am bringing this up because the information I am discussing affects all generations. We currently have an age group that was raised on hand-held electronic play toys that focus only on thumb movement, versus whole hand dexterity. This trend will continue. Amish, children play and work with their hands. They do outside chores. I am not suggesting that we go back to the wilderness; I am suggesting that you would do best to limit electronic games as babysitters. Brain development is activated by motion. The whole body is one contiguous unit, motion is life.

An additional point, that may be a part of your long-term health, is the fact that you may not get enough restful, restorative sleep. Growth hormone is released at night. How hungry are you in the morning when you awake? If you are hungry, that is a good sign that your body is actively creating growth hormone for restoration. If you are not hungry when you awake, feel worn out and only get going with a cup of coffee, you may want to evaluate your habits before you go to bed.

The Amish are able to get more restorative sleep. They do not look at computer screens or watch TV before they go to bed because they have no electricity. The stimulation you input into your body has a lot to do with your inability to fall asleep and go into a restorative state. The pineal gland, a small mass of tissue in your body, is affected by light. This same gland produces melatonin for sleep. If you are worn out and have the symptoms of Adrenal Fatigue and burnout as discussed earlier in Chapter Eight, I would suggest that you limit your exposure to the light from your lap top and other monitors and give your brain a chance to sort out the activities of the day. If you have insomnia issues, do absolutely nothing for at least one hour before bed.

Roughly about 30 percent of the patients I treat, sleep six hours or less; more than 50 percent get less than eight hours nightly. Those on swing shifts or who work nights have some of the greatest challenges with their health because their biological clock never really has time to adjust itself. The Amish go to bed at dusk or a little later and are up at the crack of dawn. They get the restorative benefit of the natural release of growth hormone.

When it comes to aging, the Amish do work very hard and it does take a toll on their physical body. However, one area that they do not have to contend with is the damaging consequences of the electro magnetic energy that is around us with cell phones, computers, micro-waves and even air travel. We are bombarded daily with invisible electromagnetic particles that you do not think about because you do not see, feel, taste or touch. They do, in fact, harm us by creating damaging effects on the strands of RNA and DNA in the genetic makeup of our cells. When the genetic material of your cells is altered, then cancer has an opportunity to proliferate. Environmental physical toxins and electromagnetic contamination will alter your body's potential to operate harmoniously; you will be in a chronic state of disease without addressing your relentless exposure to these pollutants. We suggest an herb called Rhodiola® from Standard Process Labs as a recommended support if you happen to be one of the blue tooth, computer or video game warriors.

The Amish, fortunately, do not need to deal with the negative effects of this modern convenience, and they also do not have to deal with the adrenal burnout that is a part of the squeal.

I have learned many things from observing the Amish. I would recommend that each of us create a bit of real life back into our daily schedules. I would encourage you to go outdoors, take a walk and get active. Think about what you are eating. Focus on foods that would satisfy the warming and cooling of your body and not just putting in calories. I would really try to avoid citrus all together; especially if you have pain that is relentless and you consume citrus items regularly. Just try it. I consistently get good reports. I know what you are thinking. Where do I get my vitamin C? Try red and yellow peppers along with other colorful produce such as asparagus, broccoli and cauliflower. Oranges are not the only source of vitamin C.

NOTES_____

_____

_____

_____

_____

_____

_____

_____

PART III

JUST TELL ME
WHAT TO DO

14
How Do You Exercise?

There is definitely a proactive exercise mindset and movement in America today. It also seems that there are two types of individuals: those who are disciplined and stick to it, and those who exercise for a season then fall off the "weight bench" and go home to sit on the couch.

I know the food industry is bewildered. Who do they cater to? Individuals who watch what they eat *or* others who eat in reckless abandonment? Look around. So many people are overweight and do not even know where to begin to lose weight. Any long-term, successful weight-loss program needs to include exercise as a part of one's regular daily activity. Exercising should become as normal as brushing your teeth or taking a shower; it is a significant factor for optimal health. You may want to read *The Seven Principles of Burning Fat* by Eric Berg, D.C. Each body type does better on an exercise regime tailored to one's own body and hormone system.

Motion is life. Activity creates the feel-good hormones in the body. The benefits of exercise also include:

- a proper flow of lymph fluid
- healthy stress to the heart muscle
- the piezoelectric effect needed for bone strength
- posture and foundation strength

✝ more oxygen flow for cell health

Exercise helps every structure and organ in your body.

OK, so where do you start. First, you are not going to run a marathon or lift your own body weight the first week. You want to go slow and steady, like the rabbit and the turtle tale. You just need to start! You would be wise to have an assessment and direction by a healthcare provider. You may want to have some blood tests performed that would include a basic metabolic panel with your cholesterol, triglycerides and glucose. You will be surprised how those levels will go to normal with just a bit of movement. You also are creating a base to monitor your improvement and be a part of your long-term motivation and evaluation.

You may want to find a few exercise partners, not just one or two. You will be amazed how some people may not be as motivated and will drop out for various "very good" reasons. I recently had this happen with two of my patients. One was having some personal stress and was not able to go to our local college to exercise, so the second one thought she would just wait until the first one was able. Six months went by and NO exercise by either one. I see this "losers limp" occur quite commonly.

What kind of exercise should you pursue? Well, there are a lot of options. Some recreations can be considered exercise for some since it does get your heart rate going. I want you to focus on moving oxygen. This means activities like walking, dancing, jogging, playing tennis and racquetball. That list could be endless. The whole point is movement. Movement that gets blood, lymph fluid and oxygen flowing.

The next type of exercise I would like you to concentrate on is strength training. I encourage both aerobic and muscle toning activities. I have people in my practice that jog daily on their treadmill and bicycles, but have "loose flesh" around their tummy and arms. I personally do not see a problem with exercising some part of your body everyday. Now I am not suggesting that you can never take a day off. However, I want you to know that there are so many options available that you could go a whole week and do something different everyday without overdoing one part. So, it will be your choice.

For strength training it would be in your best interest to go to a community center, exercise facility, school, church or somewhere that a "trained" professional can assist you while you are learning a routine for yourself. Now, some routines can become ruts, and ruts are graves without ends, so vary what you do. You can go to multiple locations. I know in our town, I have patients that attend three or four different venues, and each one is either free or have a very minimal charge.

You could use free weights, machines, and/or exercise bands. There is almost a limitless amount of possibilities; you do not want to overdo it. Your goal should be to slowly put enough resistance against the muscles to create tension, which will increase blood flow and muscle contractions. You will be amazed at how quickly your muscles will respond; they will rejoice with the activity.

I also encourage my patients to use the large "physio balls"; the large colorful balls that you see at the gym. They are great for improving your posture and strengthening your core. Core work is also excellent. Pilates and yoga are very good for the soft tissue structures. You have so many options including: tai chi, karate, judo, tumbling, tae kwon do. Just find something you like to do, or several activities that you enjoy, and in which to get involved. I am all for square dancing, line dancing, belly dancing, aerobic classes, etc. There are books and DVD's available, so there is no excuse!

Now, to avoid those sore muscles, make sure you are drinking enough water. Sore muscles are often a result of too much acid being built up in your body. You want enough water to flush out the acid. Also, make sure you are eating enough protein. We encourage egg white protein as a supplement with either rice, almond or oat milk. Not soy or whey protein. You do not have to use a powder; just make sure you are adding some extra protein such as: almond butter, eggs, nuts, organic deli meats and beans. I would also suggest you consume some additional Omega 3 flax oil for relief of any tendon pain, and Celtic Sea Salt®.

Where do you find the time? Let's say you have little ones at home. Then you will need to do some co-op work. Get several moms and dads together and work out the details. You may need to actually go to bed and get up a bit earlier. Something may have to go; the best to go is the TV. Now, if you are an addict and need to be amused, then you could schedule around a program or just watch the program when you exercise. You need to figure it out.

The biggest challenge I see is the patient who is extremely out of shape, overweight and personally embarrassed to put on exercise clothes and be seen in public. Well, you are going to need to make some choices. You will need to look around for the right class and organization for you or start at home. Commit to a period of time, be disciplined and get to the level you want before making your debut.

It is not easy, but if you do not do anything, then in five years you will be in the exact shape you are in now, or to make matters even worse, you will be heavier and in worse shape. The average person over forty, loses about five percent of their muscle mass every decade. When you lose muscle, you lose the ability to burn those extra carbohydrates. So the spiral downward will continue.

JUST TELL ME WHAT TO DO!!

- Exercise at least one half-hour daily. Do something!
- Start with walking; it is by far the easiest and the most cost effective.
- Drink more water if your muscles are sore.
- Eat extra protein including beans, almonds, nuts, eggs and organic deli meat.
- Vary your exercise to include strengthening, oxygen moving (aerobic) and core strengthening activities.
- ONCE YOU START — DO NOT STOP!

NOTES_____

_____

_____

_____

_____

_____

_____

_____

15
What Tests Should You Have Completed?

I would like, once again, to applaud you on your persistence to achieve optimal health by taking charge of your own destiny. The steps you have followed and learned up to this point have been focused on giving you a basis to create a foundation of long-term health for you and your family.

What we have been discussing up to this point may seem counter-culture to some of you; people do not like to change. The way our current society is focused, "have it your way," "be all you can be," "this one is for you," is all about you having what you want now, without any consequences for your behavior, eating or otherwise. Have you noticed how popular the Food Network is? Have you observed how the hosting Chefs tend to become a bit larger every season? There are consequences to what you put in your body.

Making a decision on what tests to have done can sometimes be overwhelming. There are two main factors to consider at this point: which tests do I have completed and what do I do with the results? After solving these questions in your mind you can begin the journey with a baseline.

There are many different procedures you can have completed. Some tests are often inconclusive and offer you little information on what you should do with the results. I am also aware that you can learn a lot without being overly invasive. I will describe the tests that I use in my office. I always take into consideration the cost factor since many of these are not covered by traditional "symptom only" insurance. I will tell you the common ones that I use to direct my treatment protocol with patients.

The Zinc Test: is a very easy ten second test that requires a bottle of zinc sulfate. We put two full droppers of the solution in a cup. We have the patient hold it in their mouth for at least ten to fifteen seconds. We observe the response and the look on their faces.

Generally, because so many people do not have enough zinc in their system they do not taste anything (they say the liquid is tasteless.) This is, from our assessment, an indicator that they may be deficient in zinc. We supplement them with the liquid at two to three droppers full at least once a day until they have a bitter taste from the test. A bitter sensation is the sign we are looking for.

It is a very simple and reliable test because they also seem to have other body signals associated with a low zinc profile including: large facial skin pores, poor memory, cuts heal slowly, white spots on their nails, tired, crave sweets and men can have night time or daily difficulty totally emptying their bladder because the prostate is swollen.

The low zinc is confirmed over time with a mineral tissue hair analysis. They often, but not always, have freckles (high copper—common with low zinc) and eat soy.

Salvia pH Test: is a common test we complete in our office on all new patients. The most accurate time to do the saliva pH is first thing in the morning when you first awake before getting out of bed. When you open your eyes, slip the test paper in your mouth and compare it to the color chart. In our office we do it on all of our patients regardless of the time of day.

I would encourage you to purchase a roll of Nitrizine® paper to measure your own pH in the morning. Have a piece of Nitrizine® paper pre-cut and ready to be inserted in your mouth before you even sit up in your bed. Place the strip in your mouth and observe the color. Generally I like to see a saliva pH of 6.5. If the pH is low, like 4.5 you will look toxic because you *are* toxic. You are bathing in your own acid excrement from cell metabolism. Actually, I have only ever seen a 4.5 once with a gentleman who had pancreatic cancer and enjoyed an additional five years of life under our care after he was told he had four months to live.

I am looking at extreme levels of color. If the paper turns yellow or 4.5 to 5.5 I know I have someone who is probably acidic. We do not want acid. This is a pre-destructive life pattern that, unless it is addressed, often ends as cancer. They are eating acid producing foods. See the pH chart in the Appendix. Sugar also creates an acid pH. These patients **must** change their eating and drinking patterns if they want to live a long and healthy life. Normally, they do not drink adequate water but enjoy soda, coffee, tea and alcohol.

On the other hand, if the color of the paper is purple or 7.0 to 7.5, that is alkaline. These patients will more than likely not die of cancer, but they may have digestive distress and/or pain syndromes because they are too alkaline. This often occurs because they are eating TOO MANY FRUITS. They are addicted to juices, especially citrus juice. They will often have pain in the middle of the muscle on their upper arm. This is a common finding for ladies, especially over forty, with Deltoid bursitis (pain in the upper arm shoulder region). Cut back on the citrus and try adding a good source of organic apple cider vinegar. We use an Apple Cider Vinegar product from Omega Nutrition.

Changing your diet for three months is not necessarily going to immediately change your pH. It may take anywhere from six months to two years. One other point about pH: good posture is needed for the lungs to blow off the acid. The lungs are your best tool for helping you balance the acid pH by blowing off acid during breathing. Human cell physiology ends with an acid waste product. Drinking water will give relief to those who suffer arm and leg pain caused by nerves inflamed by pyruvic acidosis due to carbohydrate metabolism.

After you have a handle on your pH level, and you have adapted your lifestyle accordingly, you only need to check you pH periodically. I would suggest maybe once a month or so. More often if you are under active treatment for some type of destructive health process.

Saliva Test: In my experience, I have seen individuals with parasites also have yeast infestation. This may be a reason why pizza/bread is "craved"! A simple test called the "Saliva Test" can be completed as a screen. Generally, if you have a positive test, you more than likely have parasites and yeast.

First thing in the morning, before brushing your teeth, or eating or drinking anything, spit into a glass of cold water. If the saliva goes to the bottom of the glass, whether in a long string(s) or bunched up in a ball, yeast may be present in the system. If the saliva stays afloat on the top of the water, this suggests to me that there is not enough yeast present to create challenges.

Saliva Hormone Test: Saliva testing is a very logical and useful tool. There are hormones and constituents in body fluids that can be evaluated. You need to be cautious, just as in a blood test, to look at the whole picture; especially noting the body signals you are having when the tests are being completed. I generally do not complete serum hormone analysis because the hormones are bound to protein, unlike the saliva hormone levels that are in a free state and give a better picture of the status of hormone levels.

I generally test for two items with saliva. I like to evaluate progesterone and estrogen. I know there are other factors that can be evaluated, such as DHEA, testosterone and cortisol, which can be very useful but, as a rule, I do not recommend a lot of "outside in" actual hormone type supplements. My focus has been to feed the body and let the body heal itself by making the hormones it was designed to create for itself. I have used a lot of the popular "media nutrients" but have found that I get long-lasting results by coaching the patient on how to eat right and let the body do its own thing.

I would recommend a saliva test for an assessment on your progesterone and estrogen level to establish a base of your levels. You can create a plan to chart a course of lifestyle that will improve your hormonal health. If you have been using progesterone creams, you should discontinue them for about three months before you take samples from your saliva to get an accurate assessment.

Armpit Temperature: Taking your armpit temperature is a simple procedure that will give you some insight into your core function. It is not specific for any condition; it is a guide and tool that I use in my practice. What I suggest is using a shake down thermometer. Prepare it by shaking it down the night before and put it on your nightstand by your bed. When you first wake in the morning, before you go to the facility, place the thermometer in your armpit. Hold it there for ten minutes. Do not move. Look at the degrees. It should be 97.8°F or higher. If it is lower than that, I generally suggest a TSH, T3 and T4 serum blood test for thyroid function (see the Thyroid Chapter (Seven) for more insight). You can use a battery operated device. Hold it in your armpit five minutes before you turn it on.

Blood Pressure: We take our patients blood pressure in three positions. First we take it while they are sitting on the exam table, second, we take it when they are lying down and third, we immediately have them stand, and it is taken again. After observing the normal sitting and lying down levels, our main focus is to see what happens to the blood pressure when going from a lying to a standing position. I have observed, especially in females, that there is a tendency to have low blood pressure when they have hormone issues.

This test is a simple assessment, or a snapshot, as to how their adrenal glands are responding. The adrenal glands are your back-up source of female hormones, especially the much needed progesterone; this is very critical for you to understand. The adrenal glands, as discussed in Chapter Eight, are significant in making all your hormones once you approach menopause. You do not need a compounding pharmacist or soy-based bio-identical source of "outside in" hormones. You need to support the adrenals and this is a simple test to evaluate their function.

Commonly, in females with hormone issues, their blood pressure is generally 100 systolic over 60 diastolic. This is low. I know you may have well-meaning physicians who will tell you the low level is great. It is not. When you have low blood pressure and/or it drops from a sit to stand position you would do best to eliminate fruits and sugar from your life. Those items are creating unnecessary stress to the adrenal glands. There is a great book for you to get titled,

Adrenal Fatigue by James Wilson, Ph.D., ND. It will help you with your adrenal gland restoration program.

Leg Blood Pressure: I have another non-invasive test for you to do if you are at a quandary with different metabolic issues. A common problem I see is leg cramps at night and/ or cramps that wake someone up from sleeping. This is often a body signal of poor calcium metabolism. Not a deficiency in calcium like one would think. Most assessments that I do in the office for tissue mineral hair analysis reveal that patients generally have enough calcium in the body. The real issue is that the calcium is not available for cell metabolism, quite a difference. Most patients scurry around attempting to get the mega calcium pill that will make their bones strong. The real answer is to get the calcium into bio-available solution so it can be useful. By the way, I do not suggest calcium carbonate, coral calcium or calcium sourced from over-the-counter digestive aides. I also will utilize this test if someone has leg cramps that are consistent, which may indicate to me a need for potassium. Drinking distilled water and, in some cases, reverse osmosis water can result in mineral challenges. It is imperative that you consume organic vegetables and select fruits, i.e., pears, plums and apples.

Here is the procedure we use. You can take this to your doctor for them to follow in assisting you with your investigation. We put the blood pressure cuff on the patient's calf. We pump it up to at least 200. If the patient is in relentless pain before it gets to 200 we back off.

Now, here is an interesting tip for you. I am sure you are aware that a nitro glycerin pill, once inserted in the mouth of someone with chest pain, will work quickly. It only takes seconds for the vessel spasm around the heart to relax. This response occurs quickly because you are activating the oral/lingual/neural (brain) route. The chest pain will be relieved within seconds, because the flow of blood has been restored due to the nearly immediate communication from the brain cell to the tissue cell.

Well, the same physiology occurs when you put an organic iodine tablet into a patient's mouth and retake the leg blood pressure. If the patient is in need of iodine to help move the calcium, making it bio-available, then you will see the blood pressure reading burst through 200 without any grimace on the patient's face. Iodine is very commonly deficient in patients and consistently creates this response. We have successfully used this procedure with a variety of products and conditions. I also see the same response with a dry source of Omega 3 fats. We use a product called Cataplex F® from Standard Process Labs in this case. They also have a product called Ovex® that will often raise the leg pressure when calcium is an issue (See Chapter Eighteen on Supplements). There are many causes for leg cramps, such as, a potassium deficiency and reduced blood flow from poor circulation, which is why you want to be assessed by a skilled, experienced healthcare provider. **Do not do this on your own.**

Twin Scales: In our office we weigh patients on two scales simultaneously that can be balanced out in the weight position so the patient can see how they are balanced. The reason we do this is because people often carry weight more on one side than the other. A postural imbalance can often result in wear and tear on the knees, hips and ankles. I see curved spines, along with bladder, uterine and vaginal challenges, as a result of the weight-bearing imbalance. If the pelvis is in a forward position, there can be a pulling on those structures. The goal of this assessment is a balanced weight on both scales, and an aligned posture, perpendicular to the floor.

Clinical Testing: It is possible to have your urine and blood evaluated for further assessment of body function. Testing is available; you may want to discuss this with your healthcare provider. Toxic overload, how your body is responding to nutritional protocols and the levels of fatty acids can be determined with today's technology. Go to www.DruglessDoctor.com for details on how we may assist you in having testing done to create a logical program for your health restoration.

Palpation: Palpation is touch with purpose by your healthcare provider. I "literally" see with my finger tips. An experienced massage therapist can also assess so much when touching a client, and this helps me create protocols for my patients. I evaluate the integrity of soft and hard structure along the spine and skeletal system. You would do best to locate a healthcare provider that uses their hands and mind as a part of their intake. Healthcare providers tend to get detached from the reality of letting the body of the patient tell them what may be the primary root cause of the problem. Don't get caught on the merry-go-round of endless laboratory testing. I am not suggesting that you refuse testing; however, attempt to locate someone who can think and see with the tactile sensation of their hands. The following are some interesting areas that you may want to have palpated.

- I generally palpate an area of tenderness on the left sacroiliac joint (found on the lower left pelvic area mid joint line) with patients that have uterus congestion with their menstrual cycle. Stimulating the area with a forceful light touch and/or percussion creates relief.

- I will often palpate the outside of the right knee in patients with chronic gallbladder issues. A tender right knee is a consistent body signal with these patients. If you have had your gallbladder removed, think back. Did you have right outside knee pain? You need Dr. Bob's A, B, C's — Apple, Beet & Carrots along with Cholacol®; see Chapter Eighteen on supplements.

🕴 Feel your wrist with light touch. Does if feel boggy with fluid accumulation? If yes, it is a sign to me that your body is retaining water and you would be a candidate for more flax oil or precursor Omega 3 foods such as walnuts, greens and cold water ocean fish.

🕴 Have an experienced chiropractor or massage therapist palpate your left neck, shoulder and mid back area. These are the most common areas that I see relentless gnawing pain that does not abate with analgesics. The pain is referred from internal organs, especially the pancreas and liver, and increases with foods that create inflammation and alter fat metabolism. These are not bad foods, just common foods that cause pain, i.e., dairy, sugar, sweet fruits (bananas, grapes, pineapple, raisins and any dried fruit). The night shades can create pain in the same area. They include tomatoes, potatoes, green peppers and eggplant. Once again, these are not bad foods. They have solanine, which is an alkaloid substance, that can create discomfort when your liver is congested.

🕴 Be logical, an experienced healthcare provider can tell you a lot by touching areas of your chief complaint.

Observation: It is quite interesting when you have someone look at you with a trained eye and/or ask observational questions. Let me give you some examples of what I ask or observe in my patients. This list could go on for pages.

🕴 I always shake a patient's hand. The texture and temperature of their skin tells me about their thyroid and even fat metabolism. Cold hands suggest low thyroid function. Dry skin can occur when not enough oil is being consumed.

- White spots on the nails could suggest a deficiency of zinc. Fungus under the nails may be a severe yeast or fungus challenge systemically or throughout the body. I see severe fungus issues in patients with chronically compromised adrenal function.

- Bronzing of the left cheek is a common body signal with an overworked liver, along with a lack of whole food vitamin E (I suggest Cataplex E®). Dark circle under the eyes are apparent with dairy consumers. Freckles suggest high copper.

- Old acne facial scars suggest a teen life of congestion of the liver, and if it was not corrected, can still be an issue.

- Large facial pores are commonly seen in patients who do not taste the zinc in the saliva zinc test.

- Skin tabs around the neck area, and also "birth marks" on neck and face, usually are more common in patients (even teens and adolescents) who tend to have a toxic diet.

- "Cold Sores" or "Fever Blisters" on the lip or lips, especially chronic or multiple frequent ones, suggest to me poor calcium utilization and stress. This is often seen with poor digestion.

- Widely-spaced teeth, thinning hair and bulging eyes may suggest a thyroid not functioning at one hundred percent.

- Do you have spider veins on your legs and thighs, varicose veins and/or hemorrhoids? These traits suggest estrogen saturation and a congested liver.

- I commonly see an elevated left shoulder on posture assessments with patients who have a passion for sugar. The sugar reflex to an overworked and stressed pancreas which is the norm today appears to weaken the shoulder support structure with a resulting elevated shoulder position on the left. Test me on this. Look at your shoulders, if they are level, eat a candy bar or piece of cake and see what happens. I am telling you, it is a consistent pattern.

- I have also observed that a patient with a dropped right lip may need potassium, and a patient with a dropped left lip may need sodium. Potassium is easily sourced from cucumbers, while sodium can be safely found in celery.

- Patients with bowed legs may need more minerals. Teeth that are ground down or complaints of jaw pain and grinding of teeth at night may be a signal of parasite challenges. This can often be assessed with a nutritional microscopy evaluation. Also, there tends to be an elevated white blood count on blood tests that check for various blood cells in patients who have quite a parasite challenge. They also tend to eat pork and sushi, have cats and generally have many health challenges that are difficult to correct.

- I also observe patients' pupils. Those who have larger than normal sized pupils tend to burn more carbohydrates. I see this frequently in my female patients who are stressed and do not eat protein and are on a low-fat, high-carbohydrate diet.

- Smelly feet is an observation of congested detoxifying organs. The feet assume the role of "back-up kidneys." Toxins need to be released. The kidneys are overworking (high B.P.) because the liver is trying its best to do its job. The liver is compensating because the colon is sluggish and not releasing fecal material. The colon is sluggish because you're not drinking adequate water and consuming vegetable fiber. And, if your thyroid is not getting enough iodine and protein, it is creating a stagnant bowel. So, your smelly feet may be caused by poor choices on your part. You don't need foot powder. Change your habits.

Acoustic Cardiogram: The acoustic cardiogram (ACG) provides a snapshot of the nutritional status of the heart. The ACG is generally used by healthcare providers that use whole food supplements. Heart tissue is very sensitive. The assessment of the sounds created by the valves snapping shut creates a mechanical graft on paper. I use the ACG as a tool to give insight on the patient's need for whole food B vitamins, liver function, mineral requirements, adrenal health, cardiac strength and endocrine function. The integrity of the heart muscle's reaction to what you eat is almost immediate. It is amazingly accurate. An example of what I see is: the heart graph reveals sharp projections on normal closure sounds but when someone has congested liver tissue, the "soggy" liver cells impede blood flow, creating roundness to the valve closure, which is demonstrated on the graph. I use the ACG in conjunction with other assessments. It is not an exclusive tool, but I gain much insight correlating all the tests discussed so far. You can go to www.IFNH.org to locate a healthcare provider in your area that has one of these awesome tools that can be included in your health restoration.

Mineral Tissue Analysis: I learn so much from mineral tissue analysis. There are a lot of companies that do this procedure and attempt to sell you their product line. I am not saying you should or should not do that. I use mineral tissue analysis or hair analysis to evaluate many functions of the body. The lab does make recommendations; I generally review them and make my own decision based on the need of the patient and other findings mentioned here. Briefly, the facility I use provides ratios of various levels of minerals that work together synergistically or antagonistically.

For example, if a patient has low sodium and potassium I assume they may have sluggish adrenal function. This is confirmed clinically with body signals of sluggish adrenal function and the common fall of blood pressure from a sit to stand position. If there is an imbalance in the calcium and potassium ratio, I look for low thyroid function. An imbalance in the calcium and magnesium ratio suggests blood sugar stress. Elevated sodium levels suggest inflammation, and elevated potassium may indicate blood sugar stress and its association with inflammation. You can see, from what I just mentioned, that there are patterns you can look for that would assist you in your long-term plan. I have determined, through clinically-based experience, that patients who have elevated and even toxic aluminum levels generally have poor adrenal function.

I have consistently observed elevated mercury and liver spots with low selenium, and a craving for sugar with low chromium. I see high manganese in those who drink well water, elevated phosphorus in patients who have poor carbohydrate metabolism, and the elevated phosphorus is a result of consuming muscle for energy. The average American loses about five percent of their muscle mass every decade after they hit forty. You know that floppy flesh under your arms? We call those "happy Helens." They are commonly seen in patients with poor carbohydrate metabolism. I also notice elevated copper and low zinc, as I mentioned previously. Cigarette smokers commonly have elevated cadmium. The mineral tissue analysis, when used with other procedures, truly can give you a road map for improved health. This information is only a very small snapshot of what you can learn from mineral tissue analysis. You will always want to correlate all the test results to give you a plan of what to do. It is not about taking something, it is about change! I do not agree with providers that do one test and suggest many different items without also looking at the whole picture.

X-ray Assessment: I routinely complete postural or standing films on my new patients. Gravity alters mechanics and creates the alignment mal-positions or subluxation that may be creating your challenges. Subluxation is real; I have been managing them on thousands of patients with spectacular results. I discussed it in great detail in Chapter Ten: Communication Between the Brain and Tissue Cells. Here are some thoughts you will want to pass on to your healthcare provider:

- I notice rotation or twisting subluxation in the lumbar (low back) area with women who have ovary symptoms including estrogen saturation. The ovaries are necessary to create progesterone to balance estrogen.

- I commonly locate rotation subluxation at the first and second lumbar area in patients who have a history of gallbladder removal. The titanium clips are adjacent to the rotation subluxation. This is consistent over 90 percent of the time. I also reveal this to my patients who have characteristics of potential gallbladder problems: fat, fair, female and forty, and especially if they have freckles and at least two children.

- In the upper, mid-back area, I also have noticed another common finding in patients with improper diet choices. The mechanical mal-position is named a patho-biomechanical subluxation. This is significant, because it is commonly overlooked. A part of the structural change occurs and is evident with a part of the vertebra called the spinous process. They have been positioned in opposite directions versus being found in the center. A true mechanical lesion or subluxation results in the spinous process shifting as a unit in one direction. This is an important fact that you may need to show an experienced chiropractor. The misalignment when corrected can open up a whole new level of improved health.

- In the neck or cervical area, the x-ray should reveal a curve that is "C" in position. The normal arc or curve is 45 degrees. When I observe a lateral or side cervical film less than that amount, I encourage treatment to normalize that position. Patients have a greater chance to have compression fractures and osteoporosis when their cervical curves are decayed and less than 25 degrees.

JUST TELL ME WHAT TO DO!!

Tests can be quite frustrating. You would do best to have the ones completed that do not require invasion into your body; a blood draw or biopsy. There may be a point where these tests are necessary; I would not suggest you start there. See how you are doing. Focus on correcting the findings to be near normal, then continue on. Give yourself time! Too many patients and book readers want everything done yesterday.

- Always perform the armpit temperature and blood pressure sitting/lying down to standing. If the blood pressure drops ten or fifteen points, then you need to support the adrenal glands, go to Chapter Eight. If the armpit temperature is low go to the chapter on thyroids, Chapter Seven.

- The thyroid panel, in the hands of a knowledgeable healthcare provider, can save you a lot of anguish. Go to Chapter Seven to learn more. If your thyroid is not up to par, the nutrients needed to get it going can reverse depression, constipation and ovary function; the three major players in hormone health.

- Mineral tissue analysis is a non-invasive procedure that tells you much about what is going on in your body. I personally have used it to help assist many patients have a plan to restore health.

- Be sensitive to how your body is functioning. Many female patients have had excessive scraping completed on the cervix and uterus which aggravated a condition. I would suggest that you get opinions from physicians from different groups. There are some who may be a bit more aggressive than others. If you do have cells that are abnormal on a PAP smear, I would wait a month or two and make changes in your daily habits. Often times, I see reversals in smears. You might think about using a different form of contraception. You might be pressured not to wait to have a procedure performed because the cancer could spread. I would suggest that you seek other professional advice.

- You may want to investigate breast thermography versus x-ray mammography. This is a tool that does not use radiation.

- Have your areas of main complaint palpated and assessed by an experienced practitioner.

- How do you look? Is your body aligned and perpendicular to the floor? This can be compared to observation assessments and correlated with postural x-ray films.

- A postural x-ray would be a reasonable test to have completed, especially in the lumbar area, when you have pelvic area issues. I normally complete AP and Lateral films of the spine in a standing position. I also use the films to assess levels of decay, osteoporosis and mechanical aberrations.

It is imperative that you will want to have someone who is experienced look over the tests, for you to get to the cause of your challenge.

NOTES_____

_____

_____

_____

_____

_____

_____

_____

_____

16

Reversing Unhealthy Patterns

I would like to begin this Chapter with an acknowledgment that there are many dedicated individuals who have passionately given their lives treating and assisting the health of patients. I am not suggesting that you should discontinue their services. I would like for you to comprehend that you are the captain of your own ship, and it is OK to search and seek options for your own personal benefit. I know from experience that NOT everything that well-meaning individuals proclaim is necessarily right. If you are repeatedly called to schedule your "elective surgery," I would run to get a second opinion from someone in another group or hospital network.

The one major area I am passionate about is partially-hydrogenated or trans fat. This man-made substance was incorrect from the very beginning. There are ENORMOUS financial opportunities and losses for entrepreneurs created by this one item. At one point, eight billion pounds of trans fat were manufactured in one year. I would like you to chew on that for a minute or two.

I have been blessed with being in a position to collect many articles and journals over the years I have been in practice. The insights I have received from pioneers in the health field are in this book. One individual that I have gleaned so much from is David Fraham, ND.

I have learned from Dr. David that there are restorative and destructive health patterns. If you can discover that the pattern, is negative, modify it and even reverse it, you will then have a very good possibility to restore normal function. Sound easy? Well it is and can be. Unfortunately, it appears to me that destructive patterns become physiologically addictive. Just eat one chip! Only one donut! The one comment I hear the most (this may be you) from patients about their food addictions and discipline denial is, "But, Dr. Bob, I only had a small piece of my favorite apple pie," as they make a small triangle with their hand.

I have consistently seen, and helped reverse, destructive patterns in patients who had some dreadful conditions; the toughest are when they have tears in their eyes. There is one such woman who has been an awesome patient of mine for more than ten years. I know what you may be thinking, "If she was your patient, why did she get sick?" There is an old cliché, "you can lead a horse to water, but cannot make it drink." Just because someone is a patient and shows up, does not mean they will follow everything I recommend. In her case she refused to drink water and loved to eat sweets.

She came into the office with tears in her eyes, apologetically looking at me, as if she had let me down, "Dr. Bob I have cancer in my body, and they want to do surgery and chemotherapy. I don't know what to do, and I do not want to have surgery." I hear that sentence a lot from new patients. Human nature is very predictable. She, like so many others, had been addicted to destructive habits and extreme work stress, and when the "C" word finally registered in the cortex of the brain, she raised the white flag, and gave into to constructive, life promoting habits.

Although she did have surgery, and her uterus was removed, she opted not to do the chemotherapy and radiation. Instead, she made a total about face in her health pattern. She eliminated cooked and processed foods, she juiced with (carrots, beets, celery, cucumber, apple, parsley and turmeric), she had colonic irrigation therapy and throughout the day she drank a measured amount of water; she did this daily. She also applied a castor-oil pack to the liver area and received additional corrective spinal adjustments to restore nervous system function. She has had several blood tests over the last three years. All the scans and tests are now negative for any destructive growth in her body.

Unknown to me was the fact that she had a coworker who had also been diagnosed with cancer at the same time; her coworker opted to go the traditional route with surgery, chemo-therapy and radiation. Her friend, unfortunately, passed on in less than six months. I do not know the type of cancer her friend had; I do not want to speculate. But, I know you are reading this and have heard the same scenario yourself, time and time again, about someone who does everything they are told and still passes on. Regardless of your socio-economic status, it truly does not make a difference . Rich and poor alike can succumb to cancer. Yes, I know early detection and treatment are preached to everyone. Cancer appears to result in pre-mature death more often than most would like to accept, and I wonder if the "seek and destroy" treatment does more harm than good. I cringe when I hear infomercial-sounding advertisements on the radio from respected hospitals that have this military-like approach to "destroying" cancer cells (as if they have discovered this new secret weapon). Long-lasting success requires changing what you are doing.

Recently, I was a guest on a radio program where the host was a fine, well-educated, financially-established individual who asked me some questions about cancer. He went on to say that his wife had cancer, and he surmised on the air that she had succumbed due to the overdose of chemotherapy.

Over the years, I have had individuals come into the office who have been diagnosed by various world-renowned health institutions. I have noticed that a variety of people have the same medical diagnosis (i.e., Fibromyalgia, Depression, Idiopathic Pain Syndromes, Chronic Fatigue Syndrome, Acid Reflux/Gerd, etc.), and they share a common pattern of nutritional deficiencies and toxic overloads.

Make of that what you will, but to those of us who study these things, understand that we are, literally, detectives looking for a pattern of cause in each case scenario. Nutritional starvation at the cellular level and toxic overexposure result in very poor health. Can you tolerate being in a smoke filled room? Would you want to swim in an outside "porta potty" tank? Addressing the underlying deficiencies and overloads is foundational to any health restoration plan.

Over the years of working with patients who have developed cancer, I've seen that these same truths apply. Individuals with a history of cancer appear to share common underlying patterns of nutritional deficiencies and toxic overloads. Addressing the pattern has proven fundamental to restoration of long-term health to the body.

When someone comes into the clinic with destructive health issues, I am not treating their cancer. I am assisting the body to reposition itself to normal function. To treat cancer means to attack symptoms…the cells and tumors. I do not do that.

Attacking the cancer medically can be a potentially helpful strategy to slow the progress of the illness while the patient's healing immune system is resetting itself to optimal function. That is why I suggest that patients maintain the relationship with their medical physician. If the situation does not progress with conservative natural care, their condition may warrant surgery, radiation and chemotherapy.

Very often, patients, who are reaching for a long-shot miracle recovery, may come in at the end of the destructive process. In his book, *"The Answer to Cancer,"* Dr. Hari Sharma, M.D. suggests that some conditions may need chemotherapy and other medical modalities before they can successfully be treated naturally, because the body may not be capable of reversing the attack of cancer on its own.

The underlying pattern of nutritional deficiencies and toxic overloads that allowed destructive conditions like cancer to develop in the first place must be addressed. So then, what is the pattern of the underlying deficiencies and overloads that always shows itself in breast cancer?

- Low thyroid function (not enough iodine in the diet to feed the thyroid)...which in turn leads to...
- Stagnant colon function...which results in...
- Sluggish liver function...which then leads to...
- Unbalanced estrogen recycling (compounded by not enough progesterone production by the ovaries)... which in turn leads to...
- Zinc depletion...which leads to ...
- Essential fatty acid depletion

These six issues are what appear to be common among the women I consult, either before or after they have been treated with a medically diagnosed condition of breast cancer.

Here is how the interplay between these areas transpires; when the liver and colon have become sluggish due to low thyroid function (lack of iodine), the body cannot break down and remove excess estrogen adequately from the system.

A thyroid functioning at subpar is the leading cause of constipation; the primary cause of constipation is lack of fiber and water. The body also needs a steady supply of magnesium for bowel function. Magnesium can be sourced daily from a mixed green salad that you can incorporate in your lunch routine.

The excess unbalanced estrogen gets stored in the fat cells of breast tissues when it is not properly eliminated. This is a key source of estrogen saturation and the cause of breast cancer from my observation. The second source is undernourished ovaries, resulting in inadequate production of progesterone. The body requires ten times the amount of progesterone as estrogen. The ovaries are one of the three organs that need iodine to function optimally; the thyroid and breasts also need iodine to function properly.

When estrogen is in a state of saturation, the body's zinc stores are depleted. Not only is zinc essential for proper immune system response to fight off cancer cells, but without it, the Essential Fatty Acids cannot be processed and absorbed. EFA's are necessary for the production of healthy new cells. (Check out Chapter Twenty-Two: Facts About Fat.)

That is one of the many reasons the low-fat diet has been so detrimental to our female population in the Western World. Unfortunately, many women have been on the low-fat/no-fat diet for years. A thirty-two-year-old mother of three came into my office recently. When she was twenty-six, she underwent a hysterectomy due to a fibroid tumor. She was now overweight, and when I said the word "fat" (by way of flax oil), you would have thought I said the word POISON. I want to point out that she also fulfilled the statistics of the potential breast-cancer pattern of being overweight, fair, female and freckled. Freckles, you are thinking? I have seen that individuals who have low zinc (which we test with the Zinc Sulfate test) will also show high amounts copper in their mineral tissue analysis. Patients with high copper tend to have freckles. The copper excess causes overload to appear on the skin. Freckles are common in patients with fair skin, low zinc and experience challenges with their mind racing at night when they go to bed, even though their bodies are exhausted. Another finding is white spots on the nails. A young man said to me that he thought the white spots on his nails were calcium spots; they were not, rather they are sign a of zinc deficiency. Memory, healing and sugar stress control are among the over one hundred known enzymatic functions of zinc. That is why I test for it on every new patient. You should get a bottle of the zinc sulfate taste test and do it to yourself. Continue zinc supplementation until you tast it.

I also see females with low zinc and high copper, which also can be tested with a mineral tissue hair analysis. They also mayhave a history of their gallbladder being removed. The high estrogen tends to thicken bile. Gallbladder removal, revealed on a medical history form or during a conversation with the patient, is an area that needs to be addressed.

You can see that zinc is a huge part of the pattern. When your zinc is low, you will have a tendency to lose your sense of taste and smell. You may always be tired because your body needs zinc to make insulin. Insulin is necessary for the movement of glucose or blood sugar into cells. Without enough zinc, you will experience the result of poor glucose movement, therefore, no fuel to burn. You will be tired. Anne Louise Gittleman; a very knowledgeable healthcare provider, researcher and author of the book, *Why Am I Always Tired,* does an excellent job describing in detail the reason why zinc is critical for the energy cycle. I would encourage you to look up her books.

Do you notice that you scar easily? If you do, this is also a body signal to me that you may be low in zinc and high in copper. There is a term called "keloid formation." This is overgrowth of new skin. I have confirmed this on mineral tissue analyses of patients with a lot of scars and high copper levels. Women who suffer with post-surgical adhesions that seem to cause more of a challenge sometimes than the problem they had prior to surgery, may need to supplement with zinc to stop the adhesions from advancing.

Zinc is also discussed in Chapter Twenty-Two on Fat Metabolism. It is a critical ingredient in the formation of long-chain fats. Fat is used by the body to make hormones. Fat is incorporated into cell membranes. Zinc's role is to be a part of the metabolic pathway. When you are zinc deficient, your body will not have all the ingredients required to do its job effectively.

Recently, a patient told me of a new term; it was "bed picnic." Now, I know what you may be thinking. It's not about SEX! She suffered silently for two years with a condition that no one seemed to be able to figure out. She was depressed, overweight, had shoulder and hip pain, was unable to breathe through her nose, and had lost her sense of smell and taste. That does not sound like a picnic to me.

She ate food for comfort. Her husband worked different time schedules, so she created a regular ritual she called a "bed picnic." When it was picnic day, she would plan on what she was going to watch in her bedroom, either a purchased DVD/Video or TV program to start the festivities. Then she would call the pizza store and have the food delivered at a specific time. Her pillows were fluffed, and the soda, chocolate and chips were nearby on the bed stand. When she told me this, I could not believe all the planning. She had been to many doctors without success. Her uterus, cervix and ovaries had been removed years ago. She was frustrated because she had missed the last two years of playing with her grandbaby and was so depressed that she had created the picnic routine that she escaped to. I know someone reading this knows what I am talking about and can relate to this.

"So, Dr. Bob, what did you do?" you ask. Well, I know you read Chapter Ten on Communication and Subluxation. This patient not only had a pitiful diet, she had an upper cervical or neck vertebra that was totally out of normal position. After studying the assessment, including radiographic films and infrared thermography, I gently and specifically made my first correction. I routinely call patients to see how they respond after their first correction. She related to me that nothing miraculous had occurred that evening. It always amazes me that everyone wants the miracle pill and/or potion and, in spinal corrective care, the miracle adjustment. However, the next morning when she woke up, much to her amazement, she was breathing through her nose and her sense of smell had returned. She was in shock and, of course, excited to her wits' end.

When she got into her car, she noticed something. Her car smelled like stale perfume. She then realized that she was literally taking a spritzer bath with her fragrances. Since she could not smell, she sprayed and sprayed until her sense of smell threshold was achieved. Needless to say, she has made a total about face in her habits. She is following a simple plan I have available for you in the You Are What You Eat Section under The Page Fundamental Diet Plan in Chapter Twenty. Do you put more than two bursts of fragrance on? Do you eat and eat to satisfy your suffering? If you do, then it is time to have a zinc assessment. Then, start following the Page Diet. Also, do you walk by or know people that smell like they have a bottle of their perfume on? If you do, and I know you do, simply and politely tell them what you just read. Do you know why? Because I am teaching you to be a detective, and it could be a sign of a destructive pattern that may end up as something very serious, resulting in needless suffering and premature death.

You should have learned that all the parts of the body are interdependent on each other. Please go to Chapter Six on the

Liver and read the information that relates to the liver's role in this pattern. Also, I have a whole chapter on proper fat metabolism for you to read (Chapter Twenty-Two). The thyroid and ovaries are discussed in detail in their own sections (Chapter Seven). We are not talking about one symptom but a whole unit of symptoms. Remember, that you are the captain of your own ship, and you get to determine the meal and activity plan for the day.

I advise my patients to limit their soy consumption. I actually would prefer women who are anywhere from twenty-five to post-menopausal not to consume it. Now, I know this may be the opposite of what you read in magazines, but here is what I see, not what I read from magazines. Soy and wheat tend to deplete the body of zinc.

Bio-identical hormones are sourced from soy, which is one of the reasons I discourage "outside in" hormones. I would rather have my patients support their own body and have its own organs make the hormones they need. You have the best pharmacist right inside of you, making exactly what you need...provided you feed it the right nutrients.

I tend to see high-aluminum, tissue-mineral levels in individuals who eat soy. You should be a label reader. You should not drink soy milk. I would rather have you drink rice, almond or oat milk. I am not sure why so many people have to consume some type of milk. You might be wondering what you could put on your cereal. I don't encourage typical sugar-wheat-based cereals to my patients. I would prefer you start your day with half an apple with nut butter on it instead of a breakfast cereal.

I have provided some very strategic concepts on patterns and destructive conditions; there are many possibilities. You do not necessarily have to be diagnosed with cancer in order to require a correction in what you are doing. You could start with a condition like endometriosis, which is nothing more than abnormal growth of cells that are out of control, because the body is being fed the wrong foods, and the detoxification system is on toxic overload. You may be experiencing digestive distress that is aggravated by eating fatty foods. Could it be your gallbladder? If onions, radishes, cucumbers and green peppers cause indigestion, it could be. These are foods I commonly see that create digestive gallbladder distress.

So many of the conditions you are experiencing are a part of a bigger picture in your body. It is not just one system. The whole body is impacted by what you do. Your breasts happen to have a very sensitive tissue structure that is impacted by estrogen overload. You don't have to live in fear, but you would do best to live in reality, and this starts at the very beginning of your life.

JUST TELL ME WHAT TO DO!!

- Start with tests that you can perform yourself. Go ahead, look at yourself in the mirror. Look at your posture, your skin, eyes, teeth and hair. What do you see?

- Take the findings you have learned so far, and start by having serum TSH, T3 and T4 testing. Then have the results assessed.

- You may want to have your saliva tested for progesterone and estrogen and treat accordingly.

- A hair analysis will give you insight into your future. It will take time for that to be corrected.

- Have an experienced chiropractor (who understands the role of diet and nutrition) and a hands-on healthcare provider assess your spine and test results. It is OK to work with your natural doctor, medical doctor and other healthcare providers. Wisdom is with many counselors.

NOTES_____ ._____

_____

_____

_____

_____

_____

_____

_____

_____

Patient Testimony:

"When I first came to see Dr. DeMaria, I had various hormonal issues. I had anxiety, depression, unpredictable periods, unexpected periods, late periods, etc. Very irregular. I had previously been taking Ortho Evra (birth control patch) and Zoloft.

Following Dr. Bob's advice, I eliminated sugar and dairy and considerably reduced my consumption of soy and wheat products. However, it was difficult for me to give up hot chocolate, and the sugar was the hardest to eliminate. Also, I now take Symplex F®, Zinc Liver-chelate® and Cataplex B ® as well as get regular adjustments.

The most obvious improvements that I have gained are that I no longer experience depression or anxiety, and my cycle is more regular. My face has cleared up, also. I am not experiencing menopause yet. However, being under Dr. Bob's care has changed my body and issues that I always related to hormones."
                                                    Stephanie Morales

17

Cleansing Protocols

Cleansing the system can be completed several ways. My patients always seem to want to do something. I have told them repeatedly that the best way to cleanse is to stop dumping in the toxic food and beverages. I do have to congratulate them, however, because we see awesome results in our practice after patients complete one or several of the following protocols. They know this is serious, and if destructive habits are not corrected, the consequences can result in surgery and even death.

I have included details of what we suggest our patients complete. The procedures may not be for you and that is OK. You may have some other type of remedy, and if it works and has helped in the past, then by all means go for it. Most of the items discussed can be purchased at your health-food store or from a natural healthcare provider. You can always go to our Web page (www.DruglessDoctor.com) for product information. Study all the information, and do not try to do everything at once.

The instructions for the Castor-Oil Pack application are easy to follow. If you have any type of skin issue, tender breasts or a heavy menstrual flow this would be an excellent procedure to follow at least once a week for a year. I have seen very severe skin issues, cervical dysplasia and a feeling of general malaise improve because of the castor-oil pack.

CASTOR OIL

Let's talk about castor oil. It may seem like an "exotic" approach to increase immune system efficiency, but in reality, it is a simple modality to improve function without potentially negative side effects. I have used castor oil in my practice since the late 1970s, and the only side effect that I have ever noticed is the patient may have oily clothes…that is why I suggest you have a "castor-oil" outfit; shorts and a T-shirt.

In many ways, castor oil is a very unique substance. While most of us are familiar with its uses as a remedy for constipation, folk healers in this country and around the world have used castor oil to treat a wide variety of conditions. Its effectiveness is probably due in part to its peculiar chemical composition.

Castor oil is a triglyceride fatty acid. Almost 90 percent of its fatty acid content consists of ricinoleic acid. Ricinoleic acid is not found in any other substance except castor oil. Such a high concentration of this unusual, unsaturated fatty acid is thought to be responsible for castor oil's remarkable healing abilities.

Ricinoleic acid has been shown to be effective in preventing the growth of numerous species of viruses, bacteria, yeast and molds. This would explain the high degree of success in the topical use of the oil for treating such ailments as ringworm, keratoses (non-cancerous, wart-like skin growths), skin inflammation, abrasions, fungal-infected finger and toenails, acne and chronic pruritus (itching). Generally, for these conditions, the area involved is simply wrapped in cloth soaked with castor oil each night, or if the area is small enough, a castor-oil-soaked Band-Aid™ can be used.

Castor oil's antimicrobial properties, while very impressive, comprise only a small part of the story concerning this mysterious oil. All of these uses of castor oil are very interesting, but the most exciting use deals with ways to increase topical absorption through the use of castor-oil packs or poultices.

Much of the current use of castor-oil packs in the United States, can be attributed to pioneers in natural healing. Time after time, they recommend their use based on reports given over the years by many natural healers. The technique is still practically unknown and shunned by most healthcare professions today. This is probably due to two reasons: first, it's just too simple. It's hard for most people to imagine that something as simple as castor-oil packs could have a profound effect on any health problem. Second, in our present healthcare system, positive results alone do not constitute the critical factor in determining whether a treatment will be accepted by the medical establishment.

Everybody, except probably the poor patient, now seems to be more concerned about *how* something is supposed to work, than whether it actually works at all. Castor-oil packs improve the function of the thymus gland and other areas of the immune system. Patients using abdominal castor-oil packs had significant increases in the production of lymphocytes.

When castor oil is absorbed through the skin, several extraordinary events take place. The lymphocyte count of the blood increases. This is a result of a positive influence on the thymus gland and/or lymphatic tissue. The flow of lymph increases throughout the body as discussed in Chapter Five. This speeds up the removal of toxins surrounding the cells and reduces the size of swollen lymph nodes. The end result is a general overall improvement in organ function with a lessening of fatigue and depression.

Rubbed or Massaged Directly Into the Skin

Castor oil can be used as massage oil, which seems to be especially effective when applied along the spinal column. If the oil is massaged into the body, the direction of the massage should always follow the same path as the underlying lymphatic drainage system.

Conditions Responding to Simple Topical Application:

Oftentimes, there is no need for castor-oil packs; amazing results can be obtained by simply applying it directly to the skin. The following is a short list of some of the more common ailments it can remedy:

- Skin dryness and flaking
- Wounds
- Skin cysts just below the surface
- Muscle strains
- Ringworm
- Bursitis
- Warts
- Itching
- Fungal and bacterial infections
- Abdominal stretch marks
- Liver or "age spots"
- Ligament sprains

CASTOR-OIL PACK

Recommendation:

I suggest you speak to your healthcare provider. You may think that a modality like the castor-oil pack is low technology, but I have seen mononucleosis respond quickly, dysplasia of the cervix return to normal and digestive distress of long standing normalize using this procedure. It works, but I would not use it without having a discussion with your healthcare provider. You are promoting liver function and it may be something to postpone until you modify your diet.

Castor-oil packs have been employed for health benefits since antiquity. Reportedly, they were used in ancient India, China, Persia, Egypt, Africa, Greece, Rome and in North and South America. More modern applications for their use are as treatments for gastrointestinal problems, lacerations, skin disorders such as psoriasis, as an evacuant, and they are used as a vehicle for introducing medications into the body. Common usage had been for improving elimination capacities, stimulating the liver and gallbladder, healing lesions and adhesions, relief of pain, reduction of inflammation and increasing lymphatic circulation drawing acids and poisons out of bodily tissues. Generally speaking, you may wish to employ them to assist your body in its healing efforts in any of these areas.

Necessary Articles (available at www.DruglessDoctor.com):

- Castor Oil (100 percent pure, cold-pressed)
- Wool Flannel (Cotton flannel should not be used)
- Heating Pad

Procedure:

- Fold the wool flannel so that it is three or four layers thick.
- Saturate the wool flannel with the castor oil.
- Place the saturated wool flannel in a baking dish and heat slowly in the oven so that the pad becomes hot, but not too hot to place over your skin. Put your oven on low heat and watch your pad carefully and frequently, so as not to burn it.
- Rub some oil into the skin on your abdomen.

➢ Lay the warm — not too hot — wool flannel over your abdomen.

➢ Cover with saran wrap or plastic.

➢ Cover with a heating pad for one hour. It is important to keep the area as hot as possible. This is why a heating pad is recommended instead of a hot water bottle. A hot water bottle cools too quickly and does not maintain a consistent, very hot temperature.

➢ Remove the flannel and wash your skin.

➢ When finished, store the flannel in your baking dish covered with saran wrap or in a zip lock bag. It does not have to be refrigerated. Castor oil is very stable and does not go rancid like other oils do.

➢ If the flannel becomes discolored, other than the normal color of the oil on it, it will probably be due to the drawing of toxins out of the body. I have had patients who brought me their cloths stained with vibrant red, yellow, green and even purple. When this occurs, wash or discard the flannel.

The flannel can be left on for longer periods if desired. A typical use cycle would be three consecutive days per week for as long as is needed. It can be done more often if desired.

Castor-Oil Pack Benefits:

Obviously, conditions known to be related to poor drainage of the lymphatic system will tend to benefit from this type of therapy. These would include complaints such as:

1. Chronic fluid retention accompanied by swollen joints and pain

2. Arthritis

3. Upper respiratory infections involving the sinuses, tonsils and inner ear

4. Colon problems like Crohn's Disease or colitis

5. Gallbladder disease

6. Boils

7. Liver cirrhosis, hepatitis, enlargement or congestion

8. Menstrual-related congestion

9. Appendicitis

10. Hyperactivity

11. Constipation, bowel impaction or adhesions

12. Swollen lymph nodes

13. Bladder and vaginal infections

I really encourage my patients, of both sexes, to use the castor-oil pack as a regular part of their preventive-maintenance program. It is a low-budget, low-tech, but highly effective system.

COLONIC IRRIGATION

Colonic irrigation is best completed by an experienced technician. A small speculum is inserted into the rectum. Water is released into the colon and expelled simultaneously through the speculum. The colonic-irrigation water reaches deeper into the large colon than an enema. The whole procedure lasts about forty-five minutes, with fifteen minutes for you to sit on a toilet to expel the remaining water. It really is an invigorating experience, and I believe a part of one's long-term health plan. It literally cleanses the sidewalls of the colon (often lined with debris) in individuals who do not drink enough water or do not eat vegetables and are heavy on grains. This procedure also will help men prevent prostate cancer.

LIVER/GALLBLADDER FLUSH

The next (at home) procedure that can be used is the liver/gall-bladder flush. It can be quite controversial; I get e-mails from all over the world because of this protocol. I am aware that the information here can create a mixture of opinions. However, I have seen this procedure work for so many, without any adverse effects. Let me tell you, you are going to be further ahead by working on cleaning out your system with this protocol than by dealing with the bad effects of ablation, hysterectomy and even cancer.

The "nay-sayers" of cleansing are not of the opinion that food or toxins are detrimental to your health. Many of the medications that they suggest are actually the cause of various modern health problems. I continue to have patients follow the protocol for the sceanse and have what I commonly call "sightings" or body excretions in the toilet. The "sightings" would be any material released from your digestive system and bowels found in the toilet the morning after you follow the protocol. The procedure stimulates the digestive system, including the liver and gallbladder. I know, from my own experience, that there are times after eating certain foods when there is, what feels like a huge gallbladder release, especially when I eat certain oily foods. It seems like only seconds and my digestive system is rumbling, and a bowel movement almost immediately follows, usually with a loose stool.

I have patients that tell me that when they follow the protoco,l they have what looks like sludge, mucous and green balls in the toilet. I am interested that the patients have had a release, and that the system had some type of discharge of fluid; I also have had patients with minimal or no response. These patients appear to have livers that are hard as a rock when they are touched or palpated, with very little activity. The liver can sometimes be felt under the right rib cage. The lower portion can also be observed on an X-ray. I bring this up because women with spider veins, hemorrhoids and varicose veins can improve their overall health by first applying the castor-oil pack once a week, for two to three months, followed by a colon irrigation and a liver flush. One of the positive side effects of cleansing is that the skin starts to clear. This is a good sign of detoxification of the system and indicates that you're getting a grip on estrogen dominance.

Gallbladder/Liver Flush

1. <u>Drink organic apple juice for three days;</u> eat as normal. Each day drink at least one full quart of high-quality apple juice. The malic acid and pectin in the apple juice helps to soften residual material in the gallbladder and liver tissue. I would eat at least one sweet apple every day, half in the morning and half in the evening. Personally, eating an apple a day for a month prior to the flush is a very good idea; by now you should be thinking about eating an apple a day for life.

2. <u>Take Phosfood Liquid</u>® from Standard Process Labs twice a day. Add 45 drops of this product to the apple juice. In other words, you are taking 90 drops a day of Phosfood Liquid®. The phosphoric acid will serve to <u>soften residue in the gallbladder</u>. Follow this for three days. It is easy to divide the quart into two pints, using 45 drops per pint.

   If you cannot tolerate that much fruit juice, or are diabetic, use distilled water instead of apple juice, or try unsweetened cranberry juice. If you use water, you must increase the amount of Phosfood Liquid®. Take 45 drops, three times a day with the water. That is 135 drops a day. Add five drops of peppermint oil each time you are make the Phosfood Liquid® combination. This will assist the gallbladder release mechanism.

   WARNING: You must follow this step. If you don't take the Phosfood Liquid® drops, don't go on the program. One woman only followed the last part of the program: the olive oil and the lemon juice (Step 3). But she omitted the Phosfood Liquid®. She passed material but was advised not do that again, because if the accumulated material is not softened by the Phosfood Liquid® before it comes out, it will remain hard and can irritate the bile tubes or ducts on the way out. You don't want this to happen. It is recommended that you follow the entire program and discuss this with an experienced professional that has helped others follow a cleansing protocol like this.

3. <u>On the third day, after the last meal of the day (before bed), mix the following foods together</u>: A cup of high quality olive oil, a cup of pineapple juice, grapefruit juice, and/or natural spritzer. Add the juice of one whole lemon (organic is best). Stir this together.

   The pineapple juice or spritzer serves the purpose of helping to get down the olive oil. You hardly taste the olive oil. (This program originally included epsom salt. But this was too harsh on most people.)

4. <u>Immediately after you drink the olive oil, go to bed for the night</u>. Pull your knees up to your chest. <u>Lie on your right side for half an hour</u>. The oil will stimulate the gallbladder and liver. These organs will not know what to do with all that oil, so they will overcompensate and throw off whatever may be stagnant in the gallbladder. It will be best for you to lay on your right side as long as you can while falling asleep. A lot of reactions occur because of the gallbladders response to the oil.

5. <u>Take herbal laxatives next morning</u>. The next day, take an herbal laxative to flush the stones out of the colon. In our office we use Colax® from Standard Process. You can take this before the program also. The cleaner your colon is, the easier it is for any material to be released. You can obtain Colax® from your healthcare provider.

6. <u>Colon Cleanse</u>. We have seen better results when patients have **colon irrigation** prior to the flush. This clears the pathway for residual elimination. We also encourage, after

your flush, to have another colonic. If you have regular, yearly colonics, I would recommend the colonic after the flush.

7. <u>All females</u> who pass any residue, including green "fatty capsules" and are estrogen dominant (determined by saliva testing) should take A-F BetaFood® from Standard Process, three daily, until their estrogen levels become normal. Estrogen saturation is complicated by a slow-moving flow of bile and congested liver function.

8. <u>Frequency</u>. If you are really sick (such as you have cancer), consider going on this once every few weeks for a few months. Everyone is different. There are no absolute rules. For prevention, go on it at least once a year. Others do it more frequently. You will notice that the material passed is often green and floats.

Protocol Options

Experience with patients completing the flush has taught us some fine tuning for better results. It appears that there is no guarantee that you will pass anything. We have reports with individuals passing a small amount of material, while other patients pass huge amounts of matter. Read the following data to improve your chance of substance elimination: The products are the ones I have used from Standard Process Labs.

> ⸙ Fair females with freckles and having one or more children would have better results taking one (1) AF Betafood®, one (1) Cholacol® and one (1) Betacol® three times daily for three months prior to the three-day program. These supplements aid the liver in "softening" and releasing material. I would minimize cooked food and eat more whole, fresh, raw fruits and vegetables (see special note below) during this time.

- Females on HRT products, birth control pills and recent long- or short-term medication should follow the protocol mentioned above.

- Females with a history of hysterectomy would get a better response with AF BetaFood®, Cholacol® and Betacol®.

- Anyone with a history of gallbladder surgery would get better results by using AF BetaFood®, Betacol® at one (1) daily, but take Cholacol® at one (1) per day, then two (2) a day, then three (3) daily, going back to 1, then 2, then 3. You need more bile thinning. Individuals with gallbladder removal need to take Cholacol®, at least one (1) daily, and for sure, with fatty meals, forever.

Special Note: Material that accumulates in the gallbladder is often the result of eating a high-acid diet; foods burn to either acid or alkaline ash after digestion. All meat and dairy products, plus nearly all cooked produce burn to acid. The body needs to stay slightly alkaline to remain in good health. The body makes acid as a by-product of metabolism, but does not create alkaline. This must come from the diet. If the diet is primarily animal foods and/or cooked produce, the body must rob the bones of calcium (an alkalinizing mineral) to keep the bloodstream from becoming acidic. But before going to the bones, the body raids the gallbladder. From the bile stored there, it removes the organic sodium (another alkalinizing mineral). What is left behind is cholesterol, which hardens. To protect against gallstone formation, change your diet. Special Note partially taken from *Dr. Frohm's "Health Quarters Monthly,"* June 2002. *Always consult your healthcare provider with any questions on the procedure.*

COFFEE-ENEMA PROTOCOL

Recommendation:

First, check with your natural physician. I would suggest a daily coffee enema, or a minimum of four times a week for the first four months of your program. Thereafter, take as needed, i.e., if and when you feel toxic or experience problems with elimination.

The coffee enema is believed to be useful in aiding the liver in its processes of detoxification, as well as aiding the colon in its activities of elimination. The efficient removal of metabolic waste and toxins through the colon is vital to the maintenance of health and the prevention of illness.

The coffee enema may be performed at any time that is convenient for you. It usually takes from 30-60 minutes, depending on the person. It is best to choose a time period when you will feel unrushed and will generally be undisturbed.

Most people prefer to complete the enema in the morning, because taking it in the evening tends to keep them awake at night or disrupts their sleep. Others find that their sleep is not at all bothered and prefer the enema in the evening.

Some find it preferable to perform the enema before a meal, while others prefer it following a meal or between meals. There is really no best time to do the enema; it is only a matter of individual preference.

Necessary Ingredients:

COFFEE — Must be organically grown. Commercial/conventional coffees are loaded with herbicides and pesticides. Organic coffee is available through health-food stores and select coffee outlets. Never use instant or decaffeinated coffees.

ENEMA BAG — Any bag designed for enema usage is acceptable. Most have found the use of the type that is designed as a combination enema/douche bag to be preferable to the combination enema/douche/hot water bottle. The former conveniently has a permanently open, wide mouth at one end allowing the easy addition of liquid, whereas those of the hot water bottle variety require constant sealing and unsealing for their use.

COLON TUBE — A 30-inch colon tube is required. The two-inch enema nozzle that usually comes with the enema bag is insufficient for the high enema. Colon tubes are generally available from a hospital supply or a drug store.

LUBRICANT — a lubricant is required for the insertion of the colon tube. Any natural lubricant is acceptable. Avoid any commercial, chemical lubricants. Natural herbal ointments are available from health-food stores. Chickweed herbal ointment can be used. Natural oils or butter can also be used.

Preparation:

Coffee may be prepared using glass, stainless steel or enamel cookware. Never use aluminum or Teflon.

Unboiled coffee using the "drip" or the "toddy" method is the preferable means of preparation. However, the use of an electric percolator is acceptable. You can also just use a saucepan: Fill the pan with a quart of pure water. Bring water to a boil and immediately turn off the burner. Add the desired amount of ground coffee and steep until cooled to the desired temperature; strain and use.

Distilled water or water purified through reverse osmosis is the water of choice. Tap water is generally unsuitable for drinking or for enemas in a health-building program.

Use anywhere from 1 teaspoon to 4 tablespoons of coffee grounds to a quart of water. Your coffee enema solution should be at room temperature or only slightly warmer at the time of usage. Too hot or too cool may cause your colon to contract, resulting in difficulty in the performance of the enema.

Coffee-Enema Procedure:

If you are having regular bowel movements, the enema should be performed preferably following the bowel movement rather than before it. When you do coffee enemas on a regular, daily basis, you may not accumulate enough bulk to continue to have regular movements. If this is the case, you should not strain to have a natural bowel movement first, as this may result in the development of hemorrhoids. When your program of daily enemas is discontinued, your normal daily bowel movements will resume. The enemas will sufficiently serve to evacuate the bowel if you do not have a natural movement.

ARRANGE AN AREA ON THE BATHROOM FLOOR TO INFUSE THE COFFEE SOLUTION.

Most people lay an old towel atop a throw-rug or folded blanket situated on the floor of the bathroom. The coffee is infused when in a prone position, so most people make the floor as comfortable as possible. Prop some pillows against the wall and use the time for reading or making phone calls in comfort.

FIND A PLACE FROM WHICH TO HANG THE ENEMA BAG.
It should not be higher than about 2 feet off the ground (assuming you will lie on the floor).

If the bag is too high, the solution will flow with too much force, causing discomfort.

HANG THE ENEMA BAG FROM THE PLACE YOU HAVE CHOSEN.

CONNECT THE COLON TUBE TO THE PLASTIC NOZZLE ON THE END OF THE TUBE THAT COMES WITH THE ENEMA BAG.

CLOSE OFF THE HOSE LEADING TO THE COLON TUBE WITH THE ATTACHMENT PROVIDED TO PREVENT THE ESCAPE OF ANY FLUID.

ADD THE COFFEE SOLUTION TO THE ENEMA BAG.

OPEN THE FLOW CONTROL AND ALLOW A LITTLE COFFEE TO FLOW TO THE END OF THE TUBE AND OUT INTO THE SINK, TOILET OR BATHTUB, JUST ENOUGH TO ELIMINATE ANY AIR IN THE TUBE.

LUBRICATE THE FIRST SEVERAL INCHES OF THE COLON TUBE.
Additional lubrication may be applied to the rectum to aid in the insertion of the colon tube.

INSERT THE COLON TUBE INTO THE RECTUM.
Most prefer to accomplish this while lying on their left side. Ideally, the tube should be fully inserted. How this is best accomplished soon becomes a matter of individually learning through trial and error. Everyone has a different colon in terms of twists and turns as well as degrees of contraction and relaxation. For some, it is a simple matter to fully insert the tube. For others, it requires patient, gentle effort. Allowing the slow inflow of solution while inserting the tube is often helpful. Also, many find that twisting and turning the tube while gently pushing facilitates its progress. Others suggest that momentarily withdrawing the tube slightly and then proceeding with its insertion can help get around "tough corners" (the various bends and turns in the colon.) Under no circumstances should any force be used. The whole procedure should be very easy and gentle. Many people are simply unable to fully insert the tube. That is all right. You should just insert the tube as far as your colon will easily allow. It usually takes experiencing several enemas before you become comfortable with the procedure and adopt your own individual means for doing it.

ALLOW THE COFFEE SOLUTION (1 QUART) TO FLOW INTO THE COLON.
The rate of flow can be regulated with the control apparatus. When the flow is completed, you may remove the tube or leave it inserted during the course of the enema. Many people prefer to leave the tube inserted with the valve left open, as it will allow any gas present in the colon to escape.

LAY ON YOUR LEFT SIDE FOR 5 MINUTES, ON YOUR BACK FOR 5 MINUTES, AND ON YOUR RIGHT SIDE FOR 5 MINUTES.

AFTER THE 15 MINUTES, YOU MAY THEN EXPEL THE ENEMA.
You should not strain to hold the enema. If you feel the need to expel before the 15 minutes, you should do so. *No straining of any kind should be done at anytime.* The whole process should be very effortless.

Exactly how many coffee enemas you use on a regular basis will depend on your metabolic individuality. You should expect to feel a sense of ease and well-being on the completion of the enema. If you experience jitteriness, shakiness, lightheadedness, nervousness, weakness, etc., you will need to decrease the strength of the coffee solution.

The coffee enema can definitely be an adjunct to your overall cleansing program. How often you decide to do it is determined on how willing you are to make other changes. I personally would not do it more than one time per week. I personally prefer doing it first thing in the morning, but you can choose a time that works for you. Caffeine is entering your body, so if you do this at night, it may keep you awake, especially if you have a compromised liver. I know there may be some thinking that the caffeine is harmful. Let me respond with this thought: the huge long-term benefit of incorporating several cups of organic coffee in your body, and the response that it achieves far outweighs the negative effects or the side effects of medication and the disfigurement of a successful surgery with loss of organ function.

JUST TELL ME WHAT TO DO

† I recommend that you perform the castor-oil pack first, then the colonic and follow up with a liver/gall-bladder flush.

I have provided you with several internal cleansing options. The sequence that I have laid out for you is the way I advise my patients to go about doing it. The castor-oil pack is a non invasive system designed to help the metabolism of liver/gallbladder function. The liver flush and coffee enema protocol puts something in the body and may cause some nausea and discomfort. I also encourage colonic irrigation as a regular biannual event.

Speak to your healthcare provider first before completing a liver/gallbladder flush. You may want to have liver enzymes completed on yourself including SGOT, SGPT and GGTP. These will give a base line on how your body could be responding to the protocol to be employed, and also how it is responding to your current therapeutic approach. Many of the medications prescribed today require blood-level testings to be completed on a regular basis for your own safety; to monitor if the medications are creating a toxic state in the body.

You have an awesome base now. Do not try to do everything in one month. This is a two-year project. Give it time. Listen to your body. If you notice nausea and cramping slow down. Always go SLOW!!

NOTES_____

_____

_____

_____

_____

_____

_____

_____

18

What Supplements Do You Need?

I am contacted nearly every day by clients and subscribers, which includes e-mails from around the world, who would like to know what supplements to take for a particular condition. I generally suggest that they improve their food choices. Part of the challenge I continually see is the fact that there are so many media-driven nutrients that individuals are consuming that create dysfunction, even though they have been told that particular items are good for them. An example is that yogurt is a great source of calcium. I have found that yogurt also creates chronic left-neck and mid-back pain, chronic sinusitis, asthma, liver congestion, bowel dysfunction and allergies. Yogurt has more sugar per serving than ice cream. Sugar creates a condition in your skin called glycation where protein and sugar combine and creates wrinkles. I know what you are thinking, "Dr. Bob, where do I get my calcium?" My standard response is, "The same place cows do, plants!" Also, soy depletes the body of zinc and can actually increase the symptoms of estrogen dominance. I encourage the minimum use of both yogurt and soy. I am suggesting this because when patients follow these recommendations, they respond over time.

The latest fad is the unnatural addition of extraordinary amounts of Omega 3 fats to many foods, creating the false sense of security that you will be healthy by eating that product. I suggest eating foods that are naturally high in Omega 3 fat, such as plant-sourced flax oils, mixed greens, walnuts and green beans. Eat a variety of organic whole foods. Do you honestly think it is logical to add Omega 3 fats to foods that do not normally have it in their structure?

I do not advise synthetic, petrochemical-based vitamin E capsules and high-dosage vitamin C. I encourage my patients to eat a variety of vegetables every day, along with apples, pears and plums. I have found that most patients cannot tolerate eating sweet fruit without getting pain and inflammation along their left neck and shoulder area. I encourage non-gluten grains and sprouted bread. I would avoid "whole wheat/white bread." It is sourced from genetically-modified seeds.

Your goal should be to eat a mixture of raw and steamed vegetables and to avoid canned and frozen foods. There are many national food-store chains that offer a wide variety of organic vegetables. Any time food is prepared commercially, there are high temperatures used to process the veggies, which have often been picked prematurely. I am not trying to make this hard, but helpful. It is about that which you are accustomed. Plan ahead.

I use several products in my practice. I encourage the following items (I am not going to give you daily quantities because that should be determined after an assessment of your health status by an experienced natural health doctor): There are many excellent companies that manufacture supplements. I do not have experience with them all. I have used Standard Process Labs products for my own personal use since 1974. They are available at natural healthcare provider practices. Contact www.StandardProcess.com to find a practitioner in your area.

> ✝ A multiple supplement — I use a product called Catalyn®, which is a whole food product; normally

four to six a day, more depending on what foods the patient is consuming.

- **Calcium Lactate®** — is an ionizable product, which means it is easily bio-available to the system. Often I see patients come in with a bag of calcium that is sourced from calcium carbonate, which is more challenging to get into the system. We use the leg blood pressure test to assess the amount of calcium lactate to be used. A hair analysis is an assessment that can help determine the amount of calcium needed. Eat sesame seeds, almonds and mixed greens for a source of calcium.

- **Protein** — is necessary for every aspect of normal function. I have observed that women who exercise on a regular basis have cysts appear on their ovaries because they lack protein. Dr. Donald Lepore, in his book *"The Ultimate Healing System,"* discusses the lack of threonine as a precipitating factor in having ovarian cysts. We use a product called Protefood®, at least one a day. I encourage my patients to eat animal products for a complete source of protein.

- **Minerals** — are the spark plugs to the body. You can have the best fuel and an awesome looking vehicle, but if you lack minerals, you will have a misfiring engine, along with no energy and exhaustion. Zinc deficiencies are a common source of low energy, according to Anne Louise Gittlemen in her book, *Why Am I Always Tired.* I strongly encourage the use of Celtic Sea Salt®, from the Grain and Salt Company. You can call 1-800-TOPSALT. It is found at most stores today, and is even being added to conventional canned soups. Also, you will want to make sure you are adding this source of minerals if you are drinking reverse osmosis water. The process of water purification will remove minerals. You do not want to create a mineral-deficient state. Go to Chapter Fifteen on Tests and explore the information on Hair Analysis and the Leg Blood Pressure

Test. I suggest that my patients use Min Tran® which is partly sourced from alfalfa, kelp and Trace Minerals®.

† **Organ support tissue** — In my practice I recommend a supplement protocol determined by the organ I have found to be a major source of the patient's issues. Conventional medical practitioners focus on symptomatic pharmaceutical care and are more than likely not aware of the following information I will be sharing with you. I support the liver, adrenal, thyroid, ovaries and brain function with a variety of whole-food supplements. You will want to be assessed by your healthcare provider before you embark on a regime on your own. I use Standard Process Labs as my primary source of endocrine restoration supplements. I generally use a product called Livaplex® for the liver. Ovex® and Ovatrophin PMG® for the ovaries. Thyrotrophin PMG® for the thyroid. For the adrenal gland I may suggest Whole Dessicated Adrenal®, Drenamin® or Drenatrophin®. I suggest Neuroplex®, whigh is a common support for the neurologic tissue. I also encourage an awesome product called Symplex F® which serves as a multiple endocrine support; I also may add Hypothalmex® which acts as a synergist for the components in the Symplex F®. There are many more items that can be used; these are the more common items that I get consistent results with. Your goal, with any supplementation program, is to create a food intake that does not promote physiologic stress. The endocrine organs being supplemented can, once again, function on their own. Sugar, hydrogenated oils and dairy will defeat your goal of optimal endocrine health.

† **Iodine** — is a critical component to your hormone restoration program. I would suggest that you have your thyroid profile completed as discussed in the Chapter Seven. A skilled natural doctor will be able

to assist you by evaluating your T3 and T4 levels. I have found that most people can use up to twelve milligrams of iodine a day. I use Prolamine Iodine® and/or Idomere® from Standard Process Labs with consistent success. Thyroid Support® from Medi Herb is a logical product to incorporate into a protocol.

- **Herbs** — are an asset to your program. There are huge varieties of herbs that can be recommended to support you on your restoration journey. A common one I use is called Chasetree® which stimulates ovary function and supports the adrenals with Licorice Root. The adrenals need to be supported along with the thyroid. Herbs for the liver (such as Milk Thistle) help assist restoration of liver function. Your goal is to support adrenal, liver, thyroid and ovary function. I do not normally recommend herbs specific for female hormones like black cohosh or Don Qui. I have found that by supporting the restoration of the organs, the body will make its own bio-necessary hormones. I know that many people get symptomatic relief using media established herbs; I personally prefer to re-establish normal function associated with appropriate lifestyle modification. Tribulus® is a great precursor for supporting overall female hormonal health.

- **Soy and Bio-identical supplementation** — If you are currently using this approach and feel confident with how your body is responding, then I would continue with it. However, I treat patients every day and get e-mails from around the world telling me about the issues they have with soy-based products. I do not consistently get positive statements because most individuals are not coached to change their daily routine; they are depending on an "outside in" item that really is not promoting functional restoration. You will need to discuss your options with your natural drugless doctor.

Interestingly enough, The Center For Science in The Public Interest (CSPI), a well-respected organization that is a *watch dog* for the public, in their September 2005 issue, Volume 32, Number 7, page 7, stated in The Bottom Line bullet on SOY, "Researchers don't know whether soy can lower the risk of breast cancer." I have read many authorities. I have not consistently read research that agreed that soy was a positive fact for women. If I were you, I would not consume soy. There is no guarantee that it will give you the effect that you may be looking for.

Note: A source of information on soy and its impact on health can be found at the <u>Soy Online Service</u>, and in particular, its page on phyto-estrogenic effects of soy, and its <u>impact on the thyroid</u>.

NOTES_____

_____

_____

_____

_____

_____

_____

19
How to Get Off Your Medication

L et me give you the real facts that I see in my natural healthcare practice. Every day, I have new patients that come into the office who are very frustrated; they don't feel good and no one seems to understand why. They want to get off their medication and do not even know why they were put on it in the first place. I will be focusing on the items I commonly see in my practice: antidepressants, thyroid medication, digestive distress and pain medications.

Do not go off your medication without first speaking to your healthcare provider; work together because this is a team effort. I have found that most practitioners today know that their patients are proactive and have more time to research natural remedies. They are aware that you understand that food can be your medicine, and medicine can be food.

I just finished interviewing a patient who, when she was in her early twenties, was put on Paxil. She told me that within three days the side effects from that medication put her on the couch for one week. She did not want to go into the kitchen because she was afraid to pick up a knife; she was not sure what she would do with it. She had anxiety and depression. She had fear and did not want to be in a social setting with anyone. Can you imagine that? Well, it is true. There are millions of

Americans, including many of you reading this, that are depressed and do not know what to do about it.

Let me continue with her story. I want to let you know, that her physician switched her from Paxil to Zoloft before she entered my office. She also had psoriasis when she came in for care. She did not experience natural spinal corrective care before our meeting. Within three months, including taking one tablespoon of organic Omega 3 Flax every day and receiving spinal adjustments, she was off her medication.

When my treatments were nearly completed she mentioned that she could not believe that she was better and more than likely would never have been able to get out of the loop of antidepressants. She did not know why she became depressed and had anxiety. This is a very common scenario I often see. Often young females enter into my office with Paxil, Prozac, Zoloft or Wellbutrin. What a combination!

If you are depressed, how do you handle it? If you are currently on medication, I am first going to suggest that you have a conversation with the physician who prescribed it. He or she may not understand what you want to do and may not know much about supplementation. My long-term experience suggests that if you do what my patient did, you will be heading in the right direction. She started with one tablespoon of organic Omega 3 fat for every one hundred pounds of body weight. She eliminated trans fat or partially-hydrogenated fats from her life. Sugar was not included in her diet anymore. She came into the office and had her spine checked for subluxation. She followed the recommended protocol and within three months she was asymptomatic. For you to get results you must make some changes. This same patient was, and is, very active. Losing weight was not a part of the problem. She exercised regularly. She needed to get OIL in her body. Your body will use the oil to create the right fat for your brain.

I have patients who come into the office suffering from cold hands and feet. They wake up with morning headaches, are tired, fatigued, overweight, have high cholesterol and are constipated. Sound like you? It is the most common set of body signals that I see. These patients are normally on some type of thyroid medication with no plan to restore thyroid function.

I generally will have them get the lab tests I discussed in the Chapter Seven and treat accordingly. A huge focus that I see with those body signals is to make sure you are taking enough iodine. I usually recommend at least twelve milligrams a day. This is the amount that females in Japan normally consume in their daily diet of sea vegetables and marine seafood.

Japanese females have less menopause symptoms and other common Western body signals (hot flashes). Now, if you are on thyroid medication, you will want to monitor your thyroid lab values with the assistance of your healthcare provider. We support the thyroid during its restitution phase with items that promote restoration. I use animal-sourced nucleoproteins from Standard Process Labs that promote proper function; you can obtain these products from a trained natural, healthcare provider. The products I commonly use are Thyrotrophin® and Prolamine Iodine® (see Chapter Eighteen on food supplementation). I also focus on reducing the estrogen and cortisol levels by encouraging reduction of sugar and cleaning up the liver. High estrogen and cortisol levels impair thyroid function conversion of T4 to T3.

I have also seen, by observing thyroid-stimulating hormones from the pituitary gland (TSH levels), that up to 50 percent of patients with impaired function of the thyroid appear to have low TSH.

To feed the pituitary, I prescribe either Pituitrophin® or Neuroplex®. I have also noticed a low selenium and/or manganese level in the hair analysis. I may use Cataplex E® or Chlorophyl Complex®. These items contribute nutrients for pituitary integrity. Patients with brown "liver spots" commonly need a whole-food source of vitamin E. I recommend Cataplex E® to these patients until the spots are diminished. I generally have the patient take the product for three months and reassess. I also encourage that they take Flax, Prolamine Iodine®, and minerals. I recommend products called Trace Minerals® and MinTran®. These are whole-food sources of food.

You should not go off any medication without being monitored by your healthcare provider or one that is skilled in understanding low-dosage supplementation. One needs to understand the role of TSH, T3 and T4.

Another common product I see nearly as much as thyroid medication and antidepressants is digestive aides. Patients often take Nexium, Prilosec or Tagament. You may have been told to take an over-the-counter remedy including any one of the many calcium-enriched products. If your digestive system is not working at 100 percent, your body will not be up to par.

You need to absorb nutrients. If you do not have enough acid or enzymes, your body will not continue to get the resources it needs. Many articles and advertisements are directed toward promoting the fact that you have too much acid. This is only half right. You have too much inorganic acid produced by the fermentation of the food in your stomach because there was not enough organic acid to process the food properly. Your stomach becomes a compost pile with mismanagement of the food.

I had a guest on a recent TV program who was in her mid seventies. She told me she had been healthy her whole life. She went on to say that she had been having GERD (gastro-esophageal reflux) symptoms for fifteen years that she had learned to live with. After coming into my office for treatment, much to her surprise, within three months her GERD was gone. We encouraged her to stop eating sugar, which depletes very necessary B vitamins used to make the badly needed digestive acids. I also completed spinal correction to her mid-back or thoracic region.

It is estimated that up to 46 percent of the population who have digestive distress, also have a mid-back strain. I encourage using the "Swiss" or "physio" ball as explained in the Chapter Fourteen: How Do You Exercise? to strengthen the mid-back area.

JUST TELL ME WHAT TO DO!

- You should always talk to the physician who prescribed the medications you are taking. You should not even think of going without any prescriptions unless you plan on changing.

- It would be to your advantage to work with a natural doctor experienced with helping whatever condition you may have without medication. Do not attempt to self prescribe.

- Follow what you have learned so far. Eat whole foods and avoid processed, liver-plugging, thyroid-draining items.

- Soda, sugar, trans fat and dairy are leading items that may be a part of your challenge.

- If you take birth control pills, you might think about seeking another option. Birth control pills create a very serious hormone imbalance in the body and can be a cause of liver distress and estrogen dominance, creating an environment for dysplasia.

NOTES_____

_____

_____

_____

_____

_____

_____

Patient Testimony:

"Before making Dr. DeMaria's recommended lifestyle changes, I had been dealing with hot flashes and sweats. I also had been taking various medications: water pill, Coumadin, heart pill, Zanex, Lipitore, Requip and Zidea. Following Dr. Bob's advice, I stopped eating sugar, which was very difficult. I was a junk food eater!

The information and care provided by Dr. Bob has improved my life 80 percent. I feel much healthier. Dr. DeMaria and his office staff are the greatest. They are always there for their patients!"

Alda Wohliber

PART IV

YOU ARE
WHAT YOU EAT

20

The Page Fundamental Diet Plan

Patients always ask me what to eat. It is probably one of the most common questions I get on a regular basis. One of my post-graduate training classes was a part of the curriculum from the International Foundation of Nutrition and Health (www.ifnh.org). They utilize the Page Diet protocol in their training. I have adapted it in my office and have found it to be very logical, and it works. We seem to focus on about eight or ten different foods and that is the extent of it. Today most kids eat only about three foods, i.e., pizza, macaroni and cheese and chicken nuggets. Of course, we cannot forget America's favorite vegetable — the French fry. Adult eating patterns are really not that much different. Few want to explore beyond what they are used to.

While teaching one of my workshops, the Drugless Approach to HRT, in my office, I noticed a very conservatively-dressed woman, who I did not know, staring at me the whole time I was speaking. I was beginning to think she was from an espionage group. I came to find out afterward, that she had been staring at me with bewilderment after I had mentioned that beets can lower your cholesterol 40 percent and help clean up the liver. She — and God as my witness — did not know what a beet was or looked like. WOW! I know there are going to be foods and items discussed in this book that will be foreign to you. Do not get discouraged! I do not expect you to make immediate changes. Just try something new; be adventurous.

This diet plan is designed to assist your body in its ability to create and maintain "balanced body chemistry." Dr. Melvin Page's Phase I and Phase 2 diet is not only extremely helpful, but in many cases essential to control blood sugar imbalances as well as all other types of imbalanced body chemistry. At the famous Page Clinic, blood chemistry panels were done every three to four days on all patients. Dr. Page based his diet plan on the research of Drs. Price and Pottenger, who showed the relationship of diet to health, both physical and emotional. The diet plan was proven true when blood chemistry panels of thousands of his patients normalized without any other intervention. Many of today's popular diets are based on Dr. Page's work. Dr. Page emphasized removing refined carbo-hydrates (such as sugar and processed flour) and cow's milk from the diet. On the following food list, notice that the percentage of carbohydrates is indicated. Dr. Page felt that it was not only important to eat quality proteins and fats, but quality carbohydrates as well.

The longer you are on this diet and the more closely you follow it, the easier it will be to stick to it. This will result in your feeling and looking much better than you did with your past eating habits. As you become healthier, your cravings for foods that are not the best choices for you will actually diminish. Old habits are hard to break, so take your time in changing your diet habits so you won't slip back into your old way of eating. However, if this happens, make your healthcare provider aware as soon as possible, so you can be assisted in getting back on track. Nutritional supplements may be needed to assist you to get back on track by reducing cravings, etc.

FOODS TO EAT AND NOT EAT —
The Page Fundamental Diet

Proteins: Eat small amounts of proteins frequently. It is best if you have some protein at each meal. It need not be a large amount at any one time, in fact it is best if you stick to smaller amounts (2 - 4 ounces of meat, fish, foul or eggs at a time). Both animal and vegetarian sources of protein are beneficial. Choose a variety of meat products and try to find the healthiest options available, i.e. free range, antibiotic free and/or organic, whenever possible. Eggs for most people are an excellent source of protein. Eat the whole egg, the lecithin in the yolk is essential to lower blood fat and improve liver and brain function.

With any protein, the way in which you prepare it is critical. The closer to raw or rare the better. Remember, any time meats and vegetables are heated over 110°F, crucial enzymes are damaged and lost. Avoid frying. Grilled, boiled, steamed, soft boiled or poached are best.

Vegetables: Eat more, more, more! This is the one area where most everyone can improve his/her diet, and it is an especially important area for you. Always look for a variety, although make the green leafy type your preference. This includes spinach, chard, beet greens, kale, broccoli, mustard greens, etc.

As stated above for proteins, the quality of your produce (fresh and organic preferred) and the method of preparation is critical. Raw is preferred with lightly steamed or sautéed as your second choice for all vegetables. Use only butter or olive oil to sauté. When eating salads, try not to eat iceberg lettuce, rather use lettuce with a rich green color, sprouts and raw nuts. Do not make salads your only choice for veggies.

Fruits: Most people wrongly try to drink their fruits. Fruit juice is loaded with the simple sugar fructose, which is shunted into forming triglycerides and, ultimately, stored as fat. Without the fiber in the fruit, juice sends a rapid burst of fructose into the blood stream. When you do eat fruit, first, only eat one type of fruit at a time on an empty stomach, second, avoid the sweetest fruits/tropical fruits, except papaya, which is very rich in digestive enzymes (fruits from colder climates are preferred), and third, eat only the highest quality, fresh and organic fruits when possible.

Carbohydrates: This is a very tricky area. Most people have one classification when, in reality, there are really three different types: complex, simple, and processed. Unfortunately, for most patients suffering with imbalance problems, almost any carbohydrate is a no-no. It is a physiological fact that the more carbohydrates you eat, the more you will want. Craving carbohydrates is a symptom of an imbalance; you can use this craving to monitor your progress. Overall, eat vegetables as your carbohydrate choice and limit grains (even the whole grains can be trouble). When you do eat whole grains, only have them in moderation, and only at dinner. If you start the day with carbohydrates, you are most likely to crave them throughout the day, and then you will eat more and it is downhill from there. Absolutely stay away from white breads (100 percent rye-only bread is the least of the evils), muffins, cookies, candies, crackers, pastas, white rice and most baked goods.

There is another dark side to processed carbohydrates that is not talked about much — the connection to weight gain, elevated cholesterol and triglycerides, heart disease and cancer. You do not even need to know the details to get the idea how much trouble carbohydrates can be.

Wheat and Grains: There has been a tremendous amount of debate regarding grains. Whole unprocessed grains can be rich sources of vitamins and minerals, but *with* soil depletion and the special strains of grain that modern agriculture has developed, it is not clear what nutrients remain. The two predominantly used grains in this country are genetically engineered and have five times the gluten content and only 1/3 of the protein content of the original wheat from which they were derived. This high gluten content is to blame for many patients' allergic reactions.

When scholars have studied disease patterns and the decline of various civilizations, they found that many of the degenerative diseases developed when cultivation of grains became a major part of their diets. Chemicals naturally found in certain grains, lack of the appropriate enzymes and the carbohydrate content of grains make them a source of trouble for many individuals. Our opinion at this time is to minimize grains such as wheat and barley. Unprocessed rye, rolled oats and brown rice can be considered on occasion to give you more variety. Some of the Danish and German brown breads, like pumpernickel, seem to be nutritious.

Sweeteners: Use only a *small* amount of raw Tupelo honey or Stevia as sweetener. Absolutely NO Nutra-Sweet®, Splenda®, corn syrup or table sugar. Although Dr. Page did not allow raw sugar cane, it does provide the nutrients to aid in its metabolism. If you cheat, be smart and use only small amounts with a meal.

Fats: The bad news is that you probably do not get enough of the right fats in your diet. Please use olive oil (cold-pressed, extra virgin), walnut oil, flax seed and grapeseed oils. (Do not heat Flax oil). These are actually beneficial, as long as they are cold-pressed. When cooking, use only raw butter and olive oil. They are the only two oils safe to cook with. Avoid all hydrogenated and partially-hydrogenated fats! **They are poisons to your system!** Never eat margarine again! Also avoid peanut butter. Eat all the avocados and raw nuts you desire.

If you think eating fat will make you fat, think again. When you eat fat, a chemical signal is sent to your brain to slow down the movement of food out of your stomach. As a result, you feel full. It is not surprising that recent research is showing that those who eat "fat-free" products tend to actually consume more calories than those who eat foods that have not had their fat content reduced (low fat usually means high sugar/high calories). In addition, fats are used not only for energy, but also for building the membrane around every single cell in your body. Fats also play a role in the formation of hormones, which of course make you feel and function well. It is far worse to be hormone-depleted from a low-fat diet than it is to overeat fat. The sickest patients we see are the ones who have been on a fat-free diet for a long period of time. Like carbohydrates, choose your fats wisely — this program is not suggesting fried or processed foods.

Milk Products: Forget *pasteurized* cow milk products (milk, certain cheeses, half and half, ice cream, cottage cheese and yogurt). If you only knew all the potential problems caused by pasteurized milk, you would swear off it forever. Dr. Page found out that milk was actually more detrimental than sugar for many people (man is the only mammal that continues to drink milk after weaning). Avoiding dairy will make it much easier for you to attain your optimal level of health and hormonal balance. *Raw* butter and Kefir (liquid yogurt), however, are excellent sources of essential nutrients and vitamins. Goat and sheep raw cheeses and milk products are great alternatives because their genetic code and fat content are apparently more similar to those of humans. However, we should still be cautious using these.

There has been a lot of hype about using soy milk and rice milk to replace dairy. While they sound like healthy alternatives, they really are highly-processed foods that are primarily simple carbohydrates. You are better off doing without these as well. Of course, Vitamite®, Mocha Mix®, and other dairy substitutes are highly-processed, nutrient-depleted products that honestly should not be considered a food.

Liquids: Water is best, minimum one quart a day, and herbal tea. Avoid all soda. I would limit coffee. Fruit juices are forbidden because of their high fructose content and dumping of sugar into the blood stream. An occasional glass of vegetable juice with a meal is probably OK, BUT water really is best.

If you enjoy wine or beer and still insist on drinking them, there are some guidelines. First, drink only with meals. Red wine has less sugar and more of the beneficial polyphenols than white wines. Most of the good foreign beer is actually brewed and contains far more nutrients than the pasteurized chemicals called beer made by the large commercial breweries in the United States. Less is better. Occasional rather than regular. Because coffee and alcohol force you to lose water, you will have to drink more water to compensate. Personally, I would eliminate alcohol.

The most important life-giving substance in the body is water. The daily routine of the body depends on a turnover of about 40,000 glasses of water per day. In the process, your body loses a minimum of six glasses per day, even if you do nothing. With movement, exercise and sugar intake (that's right), etc., you can require up to 15 glasses of water per day. Consider this—the concentration of water in your brain has been estimated to be 85 percent and the water content of your tissues, like your liver, kidney, muscle, heart, intestines, etc. are 75 percent water. The concentration of water outside of the cells is about 94 percent. That means that the water wants to move from the outside of the cell (dilute) into the cell (more concentrated) to balance out things. The urge water has to move is called hydroelectric power. That is the same electrical power generated at hydroelectric dams (like the Hoover Dam). The energy made in your body is in part hydroelectric. We just know you would not mind a little boost of energy.

EAT SMALLER AMOUNTS MORE FREQUENTLY

Eating a smaller amount reduces the stress of digestion on your energy supply. Eating small meals conserves energy. Give your energy generator a chance to keep up with digestion by not overwhelming it with a large meal (the average mealtime in the

United States is 15 minutes. In Europe, the average mealtime is one to one and a half hours. Little wonder Americans suffer such a high rate of digestive disorders!). When digestion is impaired, yeast overgrowth, gas, inflammation, food reactions, etc. are the results.

Another reason for eating smaller meals is to prevent the ups and downs of your blood-sugar level, so you end up craving less sugar. As mentioned earlier, you can overwhelm your digestive capacity. You can also overwhelm your body's ability to handle sugar in the blood. Since the body will not (or should not) allow the blood-sugar level to get too high, insulin and other hormones are secreted to lower the blood sugar. Often times, the insulin response is too strong and, within a short period of time, insulin has driven the blood-sugar level down. As a result of low blood sugar, you get a powerful craving for sugar or other carbohydrates. You then usually overeat, and the cycle of ups and downs, yo-yo blood sugar results (depression and the lack of energy are all part of this cycle). Eating a small meal again will virtually stop this cycle.

Eating smaller meals also has advantages for your immune response to ingested food. It turns out that a small amount of food enters the blood without first going through the normal digestive pathway through the liver. As a result, this food is seen by the body not as nourishment, but as a threat and you will stimulate an immune reaction. Normally, a small immune reaction is not even noticed, but if a large amount of food is eaten (or if a food is eaten over and over again) the immune reaction can cause symptoms. Over time, disease develops.

By eating smaller amounts, the size of the reaction that occurs is small and inconsequential. A large meal, and thus a large assault of the immune system, could cause many symptoms of an activated immune system, including fatigue, joint aches, flu-like symptoms, headaches, etc. This reaction was called the Metabolic Rejectivity Syndrome by the late nutritional pioneer

Arthur L. Kaslow, M.D. Through thousands of his patients' food diaries, he compiled a list of high-risk foods which is much the same as Dr. Page's.

Important Note: When in doubt, don't eat it. If it isn't on the list, wait and ask your doctor or nutritionalist on your next visit. The Page Diet Plan is designed to help you reach optimal health as it has for tens of thousands of Dr. Page's patients, many of whom are in their later years without signs of degenerative diseases, such as heart disease, arthritis, cancer, osteoporosis, etc. It is not intended to make you suffer or sacrifice. Quite the opposite is true, as you will be delighted with the physical and emotional improvements you experience from the food your body was designed to run on optimally. And what you eat and drink at the occasional party or evening out is not going to be significantly harmful to your nutritional balance in the long run, so you can enjoy it.

Lastly, as with all things that are beneficial to your health, it is hard to start, but the longer you use this diet, the greater the benefits you will realize from it. Relax and enjoy the benefits!

Each of your meals must include some protein. The easiest sources are meat, fish, poultry or eggs. (Count 2 eggs as equal to 3 oz.) Vegetarians must combine proteins carefully and consistently using a different calculation. An easy way to calculate the amount of protein you need is to divide your ideal body weight by 15 to get the number of ounces of protein to be consumed per day. This is not a "high protein diet." Like many people, you already eat this much protein during a day, but you eat it mostly in one or two meals instead of spreading it out evenly over three to five meals, If you are more physically active, eat more protein.

90 lb. IBW = 6 ounces a day or 1 ¾ - 2 ounces of protein per serving.
105 lb. IBW + 7 ounces a day or 1 ¾ - 2 1/3 ounces of protein per serving.
120 lb. IBW = 8 ounces a day or 2 - 2 ¾ ounces of protein per serving.
135 lb. IBW = 9 ounces a day or 2 ½ - 3 ounces of protein per serving.
150 lb. IBW = 10 ounces a day or 3 - 3 1/3 ounces of protein per serving.
165 lb. IBW 11 ounces a day or 3 1/3 - 3 ¾ ounces of protein per serving.

I would like to explain how to use the following food guides. The chart's basis is on the Glycemic Index, which will be discussed in Chapter Twenty-Three: Sweet Alternatives and the Glycemic Index. How fast glucose travels in the system has been studied, and the resulting blueprint that can be used as a guide is called the Glycemic Index. Phase I focuses on items that are lower in the Glycemic Index. They will affect your blood sugar more slowly, creating a steady flow of blood sugar rather than spikes that create an insulin rush. The vegetables listed are loaded with minerals, especially if you focus on organic-sourced products. These particular foods will assist your body in the utilization of the protein you are consuming.

When two weeks or so have passed, you can then add Phase Two, which has veggies that have a higher Glycemic Index number, meaning they will stimulate a bit more insulin and get the blood glucose into the cells quicker. Personally, I avoid the 12 - 21 percent carbs group in Phase II. I would strongly encourage you to only eat the fruits on the list. I have found that people in our culture have major health challenges because they focus too much on sweet fruits.

Phase I Food Plan
For Balancing Body Chemistry
PROTEINS: MEAT — FISH — FOWL — EGGS
(See Protein Chart for Individual Portion Size, Page 241)

VEGETABLES: (No Limit on Serving Size)

VEGETABLES *3% or less carbs*	VEGETABLES *6% or less carbs*	VEGETABLES *7 – 9% carbs*	OTHER FOODS *In Limited Amounts*
Asparagus	Bell Peppers	Acorn Squash	Butter, Raw
Bamboo Shoots	Bok Choy Stems	Artichokes	Caviar
Bean Sprouts	Chives	Avocado	Cottage Cheese, Raw
Beet Greens	Eggplant	Beets	Dressing – Oil / Cider Vinegar Only
Bok Choy	Green Beans	Brussel Sprouts	Jerky
Greens	Green Onions	Butternut Squash	Kefir, Raw (liquid yogurt)
Broccoli	Okra	Carrots	Milk, Raw
Cabbages	Olives	Jicama	Nuts, Raw (except Peanuts)
Cauliflower	Pickles	Leeks	Oils – Vegetable, Olive (no Canola)
Celery	Pimento	Onion	preferably cold-pressed
Chards	Rhubarb	Pumpkin	
Chicory	Sweet Potatoes	Rutabagas	**BEVERAGES**
Collard Greens	Tomatoes	Turnips	
Cucumber	Water Chestnuts	Winter Squashes	Beef Tea
Endive	Yams		Bouillon – Beef, Chicken
Escarole			Herbal (Decaffeinated) Teas
Garlic			Filtered or Spring Water
Kale			
Kohlrabi			
Lettuces			
Mushrooms			
Mustard Greens			
Parsley			
Radishes			
Raw Cob Corn			
Salad Greens			
Sauerkraut			
Spinach			
String Beans			
Summer			
Squashes			
Turnip Greens			
Watercress			
Yellow Squash			
Zucchini Squash			

☺ FOODS EATEN CLOSEST TO THEIR RAW STATE HAVE THE BEST DIGESTIVE ENZYME ABILITY.

☺ TAKE FLUIDS MORE THAN ONE HOUR BEFORE OR MORE THAN TWO HOURS AFTER MEALS.

☺ LIMIT FLUID INTAKE WITH MEALS TO NO MORE THAN 4 OZ.

☹ NO PROCESSED GRAINS, WHITE FLOUR, SUGAR, SUGAR SUBSTITUTES.

Phase II Food Plan
For Balancing Body Chemistry
PROTEINS: MEAT — FISH — FOWL — EGGS
(See Protein Chart for Individual Portion Size, Page 241)

VEGETABLES: (No Limit on Serving Size)

VEGETABLES *3% or less carbs*	VEGETABLES *6% or less carbs*	VEGETABLES *12 – 21% carbs*	OTHER FOODS *In Limited Amounts*
Asparagus	Bell Peppers	*On Limited Basis*	Butter, Raw
Bamboo Shoots	Bok Choy Stems	*(Only 2-3 X/Week)*	Caviar
Bean Sprouts	Chives	Artichokes	Cottage Cheese, Raw
Beet Greens	Eggplant	Celeriac	Dressing – Oil / Cider Vinegar Only
Bok Choy	Green Beans	Chickpeas	Jerky
Greens	Green Onions	Cooked Corn	Kefir, Raw (liquid yogurt)
Broccoli	Okra	Grains, Sprouted	Milk, Raw
Cabbages	Olives	Horseradish	Nuts, Raw (except Peanuts)
Cauliflower	Pickles	Kidney Beans	Oils – Vegetable, Olive (no Canola)
Celery	Pimento	Lima Beans	preferably cold-pressed
Chards	Rhubarb	Lentils	
Chicory	Sweet Potatoes	Parsnips	
Collard Greens	Tomatoes	Peas	
Cucumber	Water Chestnuts	Potatoes	
Endive	Yams	Seeds, Sprouted	
Escarole		Soybeans	
Garlic		Sunflower Seeds	
Kale			
Kohlrabi	VEGETABLES *7 – 9% carbs*	FRUITS	BEVERAGES
Lettuces			
Mushrooms	Acorn Squash	*Limited Quantity*	Beef Tea
Mustard Greens	Artichokes	*On Limited Basis*	Bouillon – Beef, Chicken
Parsley	Avocado	*(Snacks Only)*	Herbal (Decaffeinated) Teas
Radishes	Beets	Apples	Filtered or Spring Water
Raw Cob Corn	Brussel Sprouts	Berries	Red Wine Only (3 glasses max)
Salad Greens	Butternut	Grapes	
Sauerkraut	Squash	Papaya	DESSERT
Spinach	Carrots	Pears	
String Beans	Jicama	Prunes, Fresh	Plain Gelatin Only
Summer	Leeks		
Squashes	Onion		
Turnip Greens	Pumpkin		
Watercress	Rutabagas		
Yellow Squash	Turnips		
Zucchini Squash	Winter Squashes		

☺ FOODS EATEN CLOSEST TO THEIR RAW STATE HAVE THE BEST DIGESTIVE ENZYME ABILITY.

☺ TAKE FLUIDS MORE THAN ONE HOUR BEFORE OR MORE THAN TWO HOURS AFTER MEALS.

☺ LIMIT FLUID INTAKE WITH MEALS TO NO MORE THAN 4 OZ.

☻ NO PROCESSED GRAINS, WHITE FLOUR, SUGAR, SUGAR SUBSTITUTES.

JUST TELL ME WHAT TO DO

- I would suggest that you read the Page Diet slowly and analyze what you are eating. You will only get the progress you want and expect by making changes and following the guideline.

- If sweets are your challenge, I would suggest you focus on eating more complex carbohydrates sourced from veggies. Those items will stabilize sweet cravings. You may need to seek a source of chromium and Celtic Sea Salt®, which will also help reduce sugar cravings.

NOTES_____

_____

_____

_____

_____

_____

_____

_____

_____

21
Food Transition Guide — Steps to Change

I have several food transition charts for you to use as a guide for your transition to optimal hormone health. Regardless of all the articles you may have read on magic herbs that will control your symptoms, surgeries that will give you relief or any other special "outside in" modality, you will not get the permanent, consistent results that you want and deserve unless you change what you have done up to this point.

I often hear from patients "just tell me what to do." Often they do not actually want to hear what to do because that means change. I am sure you have figured out already that this is serious. You need to do something different or you may be facing surgery and maybe even chemotherapy and radiation.

Use the transition guides as just that: a guide for you to go through the food transition aspect of your care along with the Phase I and Phase II Page Diet. You can modify the way you cook if necessary. Keep it simple. You want quality organic food in your system. You can use the Page Diet as a plan to fit in with your Transition.

Transition Chart I

Foods to Avoid PROTEINS	Foods to Enjoy PROTEINS	
Eliminate Immediately	*Acceptable Foods* *Experiment with These*	*Vital Foods* *Primarily Use These*
Meats with additives, such as luncheon meat packed with nitrites (bologna, salami, etc.) Meat with hormones, etc. Processed cheese Processed eggs Processed chicken Raised in small coops, injected with antibiotics, etc. Pork Pasteurized, homogenized cow's milk Yogurt with sugar, and toxic additives	Meat without additives, hormones, antibiotics, etc., raised free-range on organic feed Deep ocean or pure-lake fish Nuts and grain as the source to make rice, almond milk, cheese, and yogurt Goat's milk, chevre, feta cheese (Goat's milk is very close to human milk constituents) and is acceptable, but not daily.	Sprouts Fresh, raw nuts and seeds: flax, chia, pumpkin, sunflower, sesame, almond, pecan, brazil, walnut, filbert, etc. Nut butters Nut milks Organic eggs Beans: lentils, split peas, black beans, etc. Goat yogurt

Transition Chart II

Foods to Avoid CARBOHYDRATES	Foods to Enjoy CARBOHYDRATES	
Eliminate Immediately	*Acceptable Foods* *Experiment with These*	*Vital Foods* *Primarily Use These*
Sugar: white, brown, turbinado, sucrose, glucose, corn syrup, fructose, etc. Chocolate Processed carbohydrates such as white flour and white flour products White rice Anything packaged or canned with sugar, salt or toxic additives Processed pasta Ice cream with sugar and toxic additives	Raw honey; blackstrap molasses; barley malt pure maple syrup Carob Whole grain bread Whole grain pasta Grain/Nut ice cream made without toxic additives or sugar	Vegetables: squash, carrots, celery, tomatoes, beets, cabbage, broccoli, cauliflower, leeks, turnips, radishes, lettuce, etc. Fruit: apples, pears, plums, etc. Sea vegetables Whole grains: brown rice millet, rye, barley, etc.

Transition Chart III

Foods to Avoid LIPIDS	Foods to Enjoy LIPIDS	
Eliminate Immediately	*Acceptable Foods* *Experiment with These*	*Vital Foods* *Primarily Use These*
Oils that are rancid or overheated Rancid animal fats, such as lard, bacon drippings, etc. Anything deep-fat fried Artificially hardened fats, such as margarine and shortenings	High Oleic safflower, sunflower, olive oil Butter	Raw, cold-processed oils: olive, coconut, sesame, flax, almond, walnut, avocado Raw, unsalted butter Avocado Fresh, raw nuts and seeds

Transition Chart IV

Foods to Avoid OTHER	Foods to Enjoy OTHER	
Eliminate Immediately	*Acceptable Foods* *Experiment with These*	*Vital Foods* *Primarily Use These*
Coffee, tannic-acid teas; excess alcohol Common table salt (sodium chloride) Any commercial condiments with sugar, salt or toxic additives Commercial soft drinks made with toxic additives and sugar	Pure grain coffee substitutes Not more that one glass a day of non-chemicalized wine or beer Aluminum-free baking powder Soft drinks made without chemicals, sugar or toxic additives Potassium balance salt; celtic sea salt Vegetable salt and kelp	Herb teas and seasonings Organic apple cider vinegar Home-made condiments without salt or sugar Fresh juice vegetables and fruits Fresh fruit ice cream Reverse osmosis purified water

22
FACTS
About FAT

Food is essential for life. Man cannot survive without food. Americans love food. Look around; people get together for dinners and business meetings consisting of snacks, over-processed and wheat-based foods. We are not lacking in sources of food. We have mega stores with endless rows of tasty morsels. Those endless rows are part of the dilemma; there's just too much food, and not enough time committed to burning off the excess weight we gain. I can't go on without mentioning wrong fat consumption and its role in balancing female hormones! Man-made fat modification, industrial fat alteration and media fat misinformation has created an enormous negative impact on our current level of healthy lifestyle existence. I am not totally convinced there is an easy answer for the dilemma which we are facing. People are dying, disabled, chemically dependent, surgically altered, and living in pain because of misunderstanding fat. Many a gallbladder has been removed due to the congestion effect fat had on the already overworked liver. The socio-economic existence of our current medical system of patient care is largely fueled because of misinterpretation of cholesterol and fat. The pharmaceutical and conventional medical establishment generates billions, not millions, of dollars on lowering cholesterol levels to prevent heart attacks. Research suggests that it is inflammation of the vessels which creates heart attacks versus the elevated cholesterol level. Who do you believe? When did this all start? Why did this happen? What is the problem with trans fat anyway?

Here we go! Fat can be a challenging and hotly debated subject. I plan on keeping this logical and simple. Poor fat function can be the primary reason you are having so many challenges with your hormone levels. You body needs fat for an optimal hormonal life.

The names of fats and their activity should be understood so you can make logical decisions on what to eat. Fats, like them or not, are incorporated into your body for fuel and to build cells, tissues, organs and hormones. Cell membranes are made of fat, the quality of your cells is dependent on the fat you eat or don't eat!!

Saturated fats are solid at room temperature and can be from plant or animal sources, although most are from animal sources. It has been suggested that fat from animal sources is the major cause of our heart disease. Saturated fat, whether from plant or animal sources, was branded "bad" fat. Some scientists correlated saturated fat with high cholesterol and heart disease. What is not commonly known is that saturated animal fat ALSO contains "healthy" monounsaturated fats and is in itself not bad, but only a part of a bigger cause.

Monounsaturated fats are liquid at room temperatures and thicken in the refrigerator. An example of a monounsaturated fat is olive oil. It can be heated to moderate temperatures and is what I use to sauté food. It also tastes great, depending of course on the source, on a huge variety of foods on which you would usually put butter. There is a classification of monounsaturated fats called oleic acid. Oleic acid is found in olive, almond, pistachio, pecan, avocado, hazelnut, cashew and macadamia oils, as well as in the membranes of plant and animal cell structures.

Oleic acid keeps arteries supple. It melts at 55 degrees Fahrenheit. I wanted to bring this up because you may see this classification on future food labels.

Polyunsaturated fat molecules are **liquid**. They do not get hard at room temperature and they remain liquid in cool environments.

I have evidence based on observations that I want to share in order for you to get the **Big Picture**. Fats and oils found in nature, in the raw, un-cooked state, are neither bad nor good. Heat modifies fat molecules in mono and polyunsaturated fats. Imbalanced fat eating (with either a heavy focus on saturated and heated vegetable oils) is what creates a scenario for unhealthy bodies. Researchers have only recently discovered and announced inflammation as a possible cause of heart and vascular disease. Personally, I believe the leading cause of inflammation is sugar. After studying the fats for over 30 years, I do believe that red meat obviously is a factor and the primary suspect. I do not feel that cholesterol is the main reason for inflammation; it is a part of the physiology of the body trying to protect itself.

CHOLESTEROL AND YOUR HEALTH

Eudo Erasmus the author and expert in the area of fat metabolism in his book, *Fats That Kill, and Fats That Heal*, said "There is no other substance as widely publicized by the medical profession — and no bigger health scandal. Cholesterol can strike terror into the minds of misinformed people. The cholesterol scare is BIG business for doctors, laboratories and drug companies." I just thought I would start this off with a BANG for all of you that are new to understanding how the body works. People do have heart attacks with normal cholesterol while they are on drugs that trick the body in having them become low. This is a very serious issue and I thought it was time for you to know the real truth.

Cholesterol is a hard waxy substance that melts around 300°F. Cholesterol is essential for our health but we do not need to obtain it from foods. Our body can manufacture it from simple substances which it derives from the breakdown of sugars, fats and proteins. This occurs especially when our total intake of these foods supplies us with calories in excess of our body's requirements.

The more calories we consume, especially sugar, and the more red meat and other non-essential fatty acids (soy, safflower, sunflower and trans fat oils) the more pressure there is on our body to make cholesterol. This is going to be news to you, but the more stress you are under the more cholesterol your body makes because cholesterol is the precursor of stress anti-inflammatory hormones.

Cholesterol has many important functions in the body. If it gets too low (even the low range that you have been told in the 160 parameter) it can have negative effects on the body. Cholesterol is a part of cell membrane formation. Health begins and ends at the cellular level. You don't want your cholesterol too low.

Cholesterol is used to make natural cortisone. One of the reasons you have pain is because of certain medications that are used to unnaturally lower your cholesterol. Cholesterol is used to make natural hormones for water retention, mineral absorption and vitamin D for strong bones. All are a part of the cholesterol loop. Bile acids, which are very important for digestive function, are derived from cholesterol. Cholesterol covers our skin, protects it from dehydration and protects it from foreign invaders. Finally, cholesterol is used as an antioxidant. This is like a fireman in the body.

Let me tell you a story. Cholesterol is neither good nor awful. It is necessary. Let's say that you are under stress and have been eating a bit more sweet items than normal. When you eat sweets it creates a state of inflammation in the system. Our body was wonderfully designed by our heavenly Father and He put a pair of glands in us called the adrenal glands that make cortisone when inflammation needs to be subdued.

Scenario: You have been eating a lot of sweets, are under stress and eating dead, processed food. You don't feel good and you visit your family healthcare provider who suggests a blood test. You agree and have the test and your LDL cholesterol comes back high (LDL cholesterol is the one that you have been told is BAD) and your overall cholesterol is at 220. You are given the no meat and cheese abstinence story and you go home hoping to not go on another medication.

Let's break down the scenario a bit further. The sugar interrupts normal metabolism in the body. Sugar depletes minerals, upsets the formation of pain relieving fat hormones, and creates stress on the adrenal gland to make pain relieving cortisone. This cycle continues for sometime, years actually. Your body runs out of the resources to make cortisone but your body has a back up, cholesterol.

Your adrenal glands tell the brain that it needs more cortisone. Your brain sends an "e-mail" out and cholesterol is promptly released from a number of sources. The cholesterol is being transported to help assist in putting out the fire. You see, it is a precursor for cortisone (refer back to the flow chart in Chapter Eight, the adrenal chapter; it all starts with cholesterol). Now, since cholesterol is not water soluble it cannot move through blood on its own. It needs a means of transportation. We will call the vehicle that takes cholesterol to the fire the LDL fire truck. You continue consuming foods like sugar and trans fat which cause more inflammation in the body, your body is under distress and you are tired, depressed and in pain. Your blood sugar fluctuates, you have headaches, fibromyalgia, and on and on. You are alarmed! Your LDL cholesterol is going up and you are afraid so you start to take one of the most prescribed medications ever on the planet. Your cholesterol goes down, but you start having the side effects described on the sheet of paper that comes with the medication.

Here is what is happening. The LDL cholesterol IS NOT THE BAD GUY! It is doing its job, putting out the fire. HDL is considered the good guy when it is up. The reason it is up is because it is taking the cholesterol back to the fire house; the fire is out. Here is the question. What caused the inflammation (FIRE)?

I have had patients not eat eggs, red meat and cheese for years, and guess what? They still had high cholesterol. Why? Because they were avoiding the WRONG FOODS while consuming sugar and fats that were designed to be better than lard and beef tallow. The foods people should be avoiding are the exact ones they have been told to eat; low fat is actually trans fat, which creates inflammation in the body, compounded with high levels of sugar in the ingredients to enhance flavor. The low-fat, high-carbohydrate diet was created to lower cholesterol, with the premise that there was not cholesterol in the plant-sourced oils. Trans fat or partially-hydrogenated oil is causing the fire. I discuss this in greater detail in my book, *Dr. Bob's Trans Fat Survival Guide: Why No Fat, Low Fat is Killing You.*

I have had patients who did not eat eggs for twenty years but still ate sweets. Their cholesterol never went down until they got off the sweets and started eating Dr. Bob's ABC's: apples, beets and carrots everyday. One apple has 22 grams of carbohydrates so I encourage one-half a day, along with beets and carrots.

Eating apples can lower your cholesterol 13 percent and eating beets can lower your cholesterol 40 percent. I see it everyday in my practice. Cholesterol attaches itself to the beet fiber and is released in the colon. I am not talking beet juice, but beet fiber. I prefer fresh, organic beets grated on your salad or baked at 400°F for one hour or until fork tender.

Cut the beets into small pieces and sprinkle with balsamic vinegar, Celtic Sea Salt and olive or coconut oil; bake at 400°F. Cool, put them in a sealed container, and freeze the extras. I normally cook about 10 beets or more per week. I wear gloves to prevent red, beet-stained hands, and I use a sharp knife. I eat several beet pieces on my mixed green salad every day. Additional beet and vegetable recipes are included in the Appendix.

Beets do have a side effect. They can turn your stool or bowel movement a deep red color. Don't be alarmed, that is good. Beets will also help you have a firm, full bowel movement.

I do not suggest commercially pickled or canned beets. Use fresh beets from the market. I know from experience that if you minimize the sugar in your life and stop eating the trans fat, you will see results in as little as three months.

What You Need to KNOW to Avoid Partially Hydrogenated Oil — Alias TRANS FAT!

Trans fat or partially-hydrogenated oils have been one of the leading challenges facing our society today. These man-made oils have permeated nearly every aspect of our modern food chain. They have also created havoc in the detoxifying organs. I know you have heard a lot about fats the last thirty years. Please pacify me and continue on. It will make a difference in your overall personal and family health.

By now, you, like most people in America, have been so inundated with news about FAT, that we are actually living in a FAT phobia epidemic. Confusion is everywhere. FAT or OIL is not the ENEMY. The kind of oil the consumers are choosing is the problem!! You need to make wise selections.

Well-meaning, free-lance writers are looking for information to attempt to educate the public about staying thin while you eat. The food manufactures are scurrying to find an alternative for the oils they fry and cook with, keeping the taste appealing and the government off their backs while attempting to keep the profit margins up for their investors. Have you noticed that huge players in the food industry are making announcements on changing their source of cooking oils? Do you know why they are switching? Better-educated consumers are demanding healthier ingredients. Education and the access to information have changed the world in which we eat and live.

PARTIALLY HYDROGENATED OR TRANS FAT THE VILLAIN

Ready or not here I come! I would like to take the next few minutes explaining to you in simple detail the facts and truth about partially hydrogenated fat…the villain of the day. It all started in 1873, when the first "batch" of partially hydrogenated oil was developed in Europe. The research was being completed in the hope of finding a new source of wax for candles. The American public had its first taste of mass-produced "Oleo Margarine" during World War II. I remember as a child squeezing a sealed plastic bag of white "goop" then pressing a red button that released yellow dye to color the material that we would spread on our bread with jelly. Margarine is a little more sophisticated today, but nonetheless, it is not a viable replacement for butter.

Partially-hydrogenated oil, commonly called trans fat, (and by the way, the double-named product is a part of the confusion) is made by heating vegetable oil at very high temperatures. The heating process then continues with hydrogen pumped into the container in the presence of a metal catalyst. It is stopped right before the hydrogen is fully loaded, hence the name "partially hydrogenated." The exact final result of the process is not exactly known. Trans fat is one of the by-products of the process. Full hydrogenation would result in a solid substance. Partially-hydrogenated fat is not solid at room temperatures. You are not creating trans fat when you fry food at home unless you are cooking pre-packaged foods or a commercial source of trans fat (Crisco®). Frying olive oil at high temperatures does not translate to trans fat.

Here is some insight for you.

Vegetable oil does not have cholesterol in it. Animal products do. People were told to avoid products and processes made with animal tissue, i.e., lard, beef tallow, cheese, heavy dairy cream and eggs.

The conventional medical mindsets were convinced that if they could get the public to stop eating those foods, the heart attack problem would go away. What most do not realize is that the human body makes up to seventy-five percent of the cholesterol on a "make as you need supply and demand basis." **Cholesterol is essential for our survival as a species; it is a precursor for sex hormones**. Vegetable-based fat or oils do not have cholesterol.

The public was lead to believe that partially-hydrogenated oil, or trans fat, was not fat because it did not have cholesterol. Ask people who are unaware of trans fat today and they will tell you they avoid animal-sourced fat but will eat the low-fat, vegetable-sourced trans fat. Vegetable oils are liquid at room temperature. Saturated fats are solid at room temperature. The low-fat/no-fat diet fad started. **The plan was that low fat meant no CHOLESTEROL.** This was done for two reasons:

- **First**, for people who were not supposed to eat a diet that led to heart disease
- **Second**, for people who eat low fat in order to lose weight

All you have to do is look around and see that this plan has not worked successfully. People are heavier now than ever before, and heart disease and heart attacks are the leading cause of death in the Western World. Americans have been on the LOW-FAT "kick" for nearly FORTY YEARS, and they still have heart disease!!

Keep in mind the low-fat diet is loaded with partially-hydrogenated oil or trans fat with SUGAR added to enhance flavor and taste. This DEADLY combination did not help the lowering of cholesterol like everyone thought it would. It actually raised cholesterol, and the portion of cholesterol it raised was the LDL component which is considered the "BAD" cholesterol. The difficulty was compounded by the fact that trans fat also lowered the "GOOD" or HDL cholesterol. Natural, not-yet-altered-by-man vegetable oil itself will not raise cholesterol. What happens is the twisted fat molecule of the once healthy oil causes a physiology predicament at the cellular level. The body then responds with a defense mechanism that raises cholesterol to protect itself.

The medical community and the food manufactures were, and still are, beside themselves on the reports of the LDL and HDL cholesterol levels. Someone did not do their homework. That is also why we need long-term studies before it is suggested that something, such as genetically modified food, artificial sweeteners and cloned animal products, is safe.

Fake food will generally cause an inflammatory response at the microscopic cell level. Trans fat raises cholesterol because it is one of the primary causes of inflammation. Cholesterol is being produced by the body to protect itself. Remember cholesterol is being released to make the components in the body to be a fire-fighter trying to decrease the inflammation. The medical community is doing everything it can to artificially lower cholesterol, which in most cases, is not natural. That is why we have "side effects" with cholesterol-lowering medication. The body can get confused when cholesterol is lowered artificially (See the chart on page 262). Trans fat interferes with inflammation relieving PG1 & PG3.

Today the restaurant businesses alone use FIVE BILLION POUNDS of trans fat per year. EIGHT BILLION POUNDS are used by our society as a whole. That is a lot of FAT. The major seed producers are looking for new sources of hybrid-seed sources to make new oils that will not be TRANS-FAT based. These oils, by the way, will more than likely be from a genetically modified resource. NOT GOOD!!

Let's talk some physiology; I promise it will be simple. What is the problem with trans fat? Trans fat tries to fool Mother Nature. TV advertisements attempt to lure the public with tasty morsels made with trans fat. We live and die at the cellular level. The cells in our body become perplexed when trans fat is hanging around in abundance. There are many complications because trans fat raises LDL cholesterol levels. I have listed only a few.

- Inflammation response
- Small holes in the cell membrane
- Correlates to low birth rate
- Precipitates childhood asthma
- Inhibits essential fatty acid metabolism
- Alters enzyme reactions in the body
- Decreases the red blood cells' response to insulin

There are small amounts of trans fat found in nature. Generally the body will use those molecules for energy. When there is a large quantity of trans fat, the body will start incorporating it into cellular membranes. This is not good.

My experience and study with trans fat started back in the nineteen seventies. I want you to understand a few components of the dilemma with this fake fat. When you eat a meal, your body takes that food and breaks it down. Various nutrients are needed

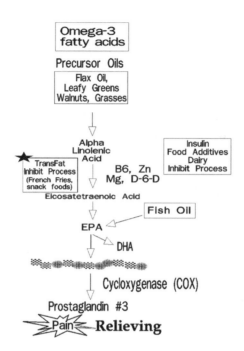

Omega-3
fatty acids

Precursor Oils

Flax Oil,
Leafy Greens
Walnuts, Grasses

Alpha
Linolenic
Acid
TransFat
Inhibit Process
(French Fries,
snack foods)

Insulin
Food Additives
Dairy
Inhibit Process

B6, Zn
Mg, D-6-D

Eicosatetraenoic Acid

Fish Oil

EPA

DHA

Cycloxygenase (COX)

Prostaglandin #3

Pain—Relieving

to complete the sequence. Items like B complex, B6, Calcium, Magnesium, Zinc, enzymes and others. All these ingredients are necessary for the body to do its job.

If one of the components is missing or in short supply the body suffers. An example would be, let's say, vitamin B6, which is commonly low in most people who diet on the run (you can see B6 in the chart), either by choice or by eating anti-vitamins like sugar. When you don't have enough B6 you can develop carpal-tunnel or wrist-pain symptoms. The carpal-tunnel condition is caused (in most cases not excluding other structural reasons) by a lack of vitamin B6. The body does not create enough of a fat-tissue hormone, called a prostaglandin, without the B6. The prostaglandin in this case is created to take away inflammation. All of this is a result of poor fat metabolism, which means you can have PAIN. It is more than repetitive stress. Think about this; "Rosie the Riveter" was building planes and ships during World

War II using manual tools and did not have carpal tunnel. Rosie had a different diet than we do today. Her meals were not convenience foods loaded with trans fat.

This next piece of information will be the most important for you. TRANS FAT interferes with the metabolic pathways that have to do with brain (DHA in the chart) and heart health (EPA in the chart). **Trans fat sabotages the process.** You can also slow and stop the progression of this process with lack of nutrients.

What you might not know is the fact that trans fat has a half-life. What is that you ask? Remember in Biology and Chemistry, uranium and other metals had a half-life of thousands of years? Well, trans fat's half-life is 51 days (which is also the reason convenience foods have a long shelf life). That means if you eat a food with trans fat or partially-hydrogenated fat today, its negative effect will linger in you, with twenty-five percent of its negative potency, for at least 102 days, maybe more. Now you can see how insidiously it affects your health.

It is estimated that nearly 30 percent of AMERICA's youth, between four and nineteen-years-old, will eat at a fast food restaurant today. The most common food requested while dining out is chicken nuggets, followed by America's most popular vegetable…the French fry. It is also reported that 30 percent of our family meals are outside the home, and more meals than ever are being ordered as carry out. With those statistics in mind, some of you reading this have more than likely had trans fat or partially-hydrogenated oils that last three months in your body, unless, of course, you are a part of the public who is educated on health concerns, and you are a label reader who avoids trans fat.

Trans fat is the leading cause of health problems today; because it has mysteriously gone undetected for nearly 40 years and has permeated nearly every fabric of our food chain. It cunningly slows and stops fat metabolism and our public is just now finding out about it. Denmark outlawed it years ago. There are major health-food store chains that will not allow it in their stores…that should tell you something.

You need to be a label reader. In January, 2006, the government required all foods to have the amount of trans fat placed on the package, but there is a loophole in this; if a product has one-half gram or less of trans fat per SERVING, a manufacturer can legally say "0 Grams Trans Fat." When you see "0" on the label, you should turn the package over and look in the Nutrition Facts Box. If you see partially-hydrogenated oils, gently put the package down.

I will give you an example of eating "0 Grams Trans Fat": eat 15 potato chips in a bag labeled "0 Grams Trans Fat" and you think you are OK. What happens at number 16? BUSTED!! One-fourth of a donut, one-half of a commercial-grade peanut butter and jelly sandwich, one delicious chocolate chip cookie will put you over the TOP. Start looking for the words partially-hydrogenated fats. They are in vitamins, candy, bread, cereal, novelty items…literally everywhere. You must become label savvy. You will be seeing more cities voting to get trans fat out of restaurants. There was a study released in the late nineteen nineties that said if you ate more than one gram of trans fat a day, you would increase your chance of cardiovascular disease by 20 percent. This information was released over ten years ago. Have you heard about it?

Let me close with this. We should not only want trans fat out of the restaurants and convenience foods; we need trans fat out of the school lunches. Feeding kids trans fat food leads to obesity and, from my research, the number one cause of ADHD is TRANS FAT. Join me; write letters to your school board and raise your voice at school meetings. The health-educated public like yourselves needs to support this grassroots drive to get rid of trans fat.

I am over 50. I needed to upgrade my life insurance policy, a common procedure in my age bracket. I have been doing exactly what I've told you to do in this book. I do not eat sweets; I do not drink alcohol; I do not drink soda; I do eat eggs and red meat (once a week); I exercise everyday; I eat a one-half an apple every day and beets at lunch with five or six baby carrots. The results from my insurance exam were so overwhelmingly healthy that they LOWERED, yes, you read it right, they LOWERED my premium. My cholesterol, blood sugar, blood pressure, pulse rate and EKG were all within normal. This can happen to you. You need to follow the natural principles that you have been reading in the book. My patients have the same results.

JUST TELL ME WHAT TO DO!!

- Fat is necessary for life, so eat the right kinds of fat.

- I would avoid saturated fat sourced from animals and keep red meat to a minimum.

- Avoid all man-made, processed fat. That would include partially-hydrogenated fats (trans fat) from any source.

- Become label savvy; I personally avoid soy oil-based products.

- Use rice oil for high-temperature frying. I also suggest coconut oil; I know it is saturated, from a plant source but it's okay. Butter, ghee, high oleic safflower and sunflower oils can be heated to high temperatures. When the oil is smoking the temperature is too high.

- Sauté foods with olive oil.

- I prefer my patients to use one tablespoon of flax oil from an organic source per one hundred pounds of body weight daily. Some healthcare providers suggest marine sources of Omega 3 fats. I am not opposed to that, but I have found from experience that you can obtain the results you are seeking by using plant-based flax oil and supplementing with whole-food zinc, magnesium and calcium and whole-food B vitamins. These constituents help create an adequate formation of long-chain fats needed for optimal health.

- ♦ You may want to try primrose oil, which is an Omega 6 oil, but I have found it would be better to use Black Currant Seed oil, which has a wider spectrum of oil.

- ♦ Oil is necessary for hormone production. Avoid all man-made fats. Especially new ones that will be developed to be "safe" and trans fat free.

- ♦ For more details on fat, including the Omega 3 and 6 classification and the different effects they can create in the body, including ADHD, Alzheimer's and Pain syndromes, you can read, *"Dr. Bob's Trans Fat Survival Guide: Why No Fat, Low Fat and Trans Fat are Killing You!"*

NOTES_____

_____

_____

_____

_____

_____

_____

_____

_____

Patient Testimony:

"When I first came to see Dr. Bob, I had cysts and a lot of pressure and discomfort around my monthly period. I had been taking over-the-counter medications such as Midol and aspirin. After following his recommendations, I now consume very little sugar, less carbs and I am trying to stay away from trans fat (but haven't mastered this yet). I now have no symptoms, not even cramps, and I'm not taking any medication!

The care and information provided by Dr. DeMaria has improved my life greatly. I have more energy, and I don't get sick hardly at all. Even when others get so sick they have to miss work, I don't get sick at all. Dr. Bob is great! He really knows his stuff and can help most of the medical problems we have today. A really great blessing and valuable asset!"
Rebecca Szilagyi

Study finds link between fries and breast cancer

A study examining the role childhood diet plays in breast cancer has found an association between eating French fries regularly during the preschool years and developing breast cancer as an adult.

Each weekly serving of French fries girls consumed between ages 3 and 5 increased their risk of developing breast cancer as adults by 27 percent, according to researchers at Brigham and Women's Hospital and the Harvard School of Public Health.

The association was not found with potatoes prepared in other ways.

The finding is the first of its kind and must be confirmed by other studies, said lead author Karin Michels, an associate professor at Harvard Medical School and clinical epidemiologist at Brigham and Women's Hospital in Boston.

"This is something nobody's really looked at before. It's really new," she said, adding, "It could be due to chance."

The finding of a correlation between French fries and breast cancer does not necessarily point to a cause-and-effect relationship between the two, however.

Michels speculated the French fries may be implicated in breast cancer because they are prepared in fats that are high in harmful trans-fatty acids and saturated fat.

The dietary survey examined the childhood eating habits of participants in the Harvard Nurses' Health Study. To obtain information about what adult women had eaten as preschoolers, the researchers asked the mothers of participants in the nurses' study to fill out questionnaires asking how often their daughters had eaten 30 different food items.

The researchers analyzed data gathered in 1993 from 582 participants with breast cancer and 1,569 women without breast cancer. The participants were born between 1921 and 1965, so their mothers were being asked to recall information from decades earlier.

Michels noted these recollections may have been unreliable, especially when made by mothers who already knew their daughters had breast cancer.

Consumption of whole milk was associated with a slightly decreased risk of breast cancer, though most of the milk consumed during those decades was whole milk, Michels said.

"Only one food so distinctly stood out as being associated with breast cancer risk," Michels said, and that was the French fries.

She said dietary influences may be more significant during early life than during adulthood, because the breast of a girl or infant is more susceptible to environmental influences than the breast of a mature woman.

Dr. Larry Norton, deputy physician in chief of the breast cancer program at Memorial Sloan-Kettering Cancer Center in New York, warned against over-interpreting the results.

"I wouldn't go out and change Americans' dietary habits on the basis of this, but it's certainly worth pursuing the hypothesis with additional research," he said.

Michels said her study doesn't prove that giving up French fries will protect against breast cancer.

But with child obesity rates rising, she said, "There are numerous reasons to avoid French fries."

Sweet Alternatives and the Glycemic Index

WHAT SWEETS ARE SAFE FOR YOU!

I would like to add information on what you should be doing about sugar. I have come to the conclusion that the addiction to sugar is one of the leading causes of so many health challenges in our society today. Men and women, once they get the physiology of the body used to eating sugar, it is like ingesting a drug that is similar to a fire that is constantly consuming. The following informationwill give you an idea of what sweet items to use.

Sugar is by far one of the most misunderstood factors that affect the health of the Western world. Either people are in denial about their addiction to sugar or are totally ignorant about how the body is paralyzed by its detrimental effects. Splenda® is marketed by saying it is sourced from a natural product; sugar. Their whole marketing campaign is based on the fact that their product is naturally sourced, and the public has bought it hook, line and sinker. Splenda® is basically chlorinated sugar. You are actually consuming herbicide sugar when you eat it. There is a battle going on between the "fake" sugars and Splenda® because Splenda® is marketing the fact that it can be heated, therefore it is safe to bake and cook with. In other words, they are saying they have the safest product. I know that after the long-term use of Splenda®, Aspartame®, Acesulfame potassium® as well as other sugar substitutes, the public will suffer with some type of severe toxic effects. I see the results in my practice daily.

I have included several examples of what I would consider possible ways to sweeten the foods and beverages you enjoy. I have also added a list of products that are not helpful to you—these are to be avoided.

STAR SWEETENERS

The Best of the Naturals

Become sugar-savvy! The term "natural," as applied to sweeteners, can mean many things. The sweeteners recommended below will provide you with steady energy because they take a long time to digest. Natural choices offer rich flavors, vitamins and minerals, without the ups and downs of refined sugars.

Sugar substitutes were actually the natural sweeteners of days past, especially honey and maple syrup. Stay away from all man-made, artificial sweeteners and the "sugar alcohols" (names ending in "ol"). In health-food stores, be alert for sugars disguised as "evaporated cane juice" or "cane juice crystals." These can still cause problems, regardless what the health-food store manager tells you. My patients have seen huge improvements by changing their sugar choices.

Brown rice syrup. Your bloodstream absorbs this balanced syrup, high in maltose and complex carbohydrates, slowly and steadily. Brown rice syrup is a natural for baked goods and hot drinks: it adds subtle sweetness and a rich, butterscotch-like flavor. To get sweetness from starchy brown rice, the magic ingredients are enzymes, but the actual process varies depending on the syrup manufacturer. "Malted" syrups use whole, sprouted barley to create a balanced sweetener. Choose these syrups to make tastier muffins and cakes. Cheaper, sweeter rice syrups use isolated enzymes and are a bit harder on blood-sugar levels. For a healthy treat, drizzle gently-heated rice syrup over popcorn to make natural caramel corn! Store in a cool, dry place.

Barley malt syrup. This sweetener is made much like rice syrup, but it uses sprouted barley to turn grain starches into a complex sweetener that is digested slowly. Use barley malt syrup to add molasses-like flavor and light sweetness to beans, cookies, muffins and cakes. Store in cool, dry place.

Amasake is an ancient, Oriental whole-grain sweetener made from cultured brown rice. It has a thick, pudding-like consistency. Baked goods benefit from amasake's subtle sweetness, moisture and leavening power.

Stevia is a sweet South American herb that has been safely used by many cultures for centuries. Extensive scientific studies back up these ancient claims to safety. However, the FDA has approved it only when labeled as a dietary supplement, not as a sweetener. Advocates consider stevia to be one of the healthiest sweeteners as well as a tonic for healing skin. Stevia is 150 to 400 times sweeter than white sugar, has no calories and can actually regulate blood-sugar levels. Unrefined stevia has a molasses-like flavor; refined stevia (popular in Japan) has less flavor and nutrients.

Fruitsource®. This brand-name sweetener combines the sweetness of grape juice concentrate with the complex carbohydrates of brown-rice syrup. FruitSource® is light amber in color and 80 percent as sweet as white sugar. Liquid *Plus*, a similar product, better matches the sweetness of white sugar. Look for FruitSource® in liquid and granulated form. Whichever form you choose, the options are better for your blood sugar than refined sugar!

Whole fruit. For baking, try fruit purees, dried fruit and cooked fruit sauces or butters. The less water remaining in a fruit, the more concentrated its flavor and sugar content. You'll find fiber and naturally balanced nutrients in whole fruits like apples, bananas and apricots. To add mild sweetness and moisture to baked goods, mix in the magic of mashed winter squashes, sweet potatoes and carrots!

Fructose in whole foods provides balanced energy.

Honey. It takes one bee an entire lifetime to produce a single tablespoon of honey from flower nectar. But that small amount goes a long way! Honey is mostly made of glucose and fructose and is up to twice as sweet as white sugar. Honey enters the bloodstream rapidly. Look for raw honey, which still contains some vitamins, minerals, enzymes and pollen. Honeys vary in color (according to their flower source) and range in strength from mild clover to strong orange blossom. A benefit of eating honey produced in your geographical region is that it may reduce hay fever and allergy symptoms by bolstering your natural immunity.

Maltose is the primary sugar in brown rice and barley malt syrups. Maltose is a complex sugar that is digested slowly. It is the sugar with "staying power."

Maple syrup. It takes about 10 gallons of maple sap to produce one gallon of maple syrup. Like honey, a little goes a long way. Maple syrup is roughly 65 percent sucrose and contains small amounts of trace minerals. Maple syrup has a rich taste and is absorbed fairly quickly into the bloodstream. Select real maple syrup that has no added corn syrup. Also, look for syrups that come from organic producers who don't use formaldehyde to prolong sap flow. Grade A syrups come from the first tapping: they range in color from light to dark amber. Grade B syrups come from the last tapping; they have more minerals and a stronger flavor and color.

Date sugar. This sweetener is made from dried, ground dates, is light brown and has a sugary texture. Date sugar retains many naturally-occurring vitamins and minerals, is 65 percent sucrose and has a fairly rapid effect on blood sugar. Use it for baking in place of brown sugar, but reduce your baking time or temperature in order to prevent premature browning. Store in a cool, dry place.

Concentrated fruit juice. All concentrates are not created equally. Highly-refined juice sweeteners are labeled "modified." These sweeteners, similar to white sugar, have lost both their fruit flavor and their nutrients. Better choices are fruit concentrates that have been evaporated in a vacuum. These retain rich fruit flavors and aromas along with many vitamins and minerals. Carefully read labels on cereal, cookie, jelly and beverage containers, then choose products with the highest percentage of real fruit juice. Beware of white grape juice concentrates that aren't organic; their pesticide residues can be high!

Blackstrap molasses. Molasses, a by-product of sugar production, is a highly-processed simple sugar that enters the bloodstream rapidly. Molasses may also contain chemical residues associated with the growing and refining of white sugar. If you grew up on conventional molasses, your taste buds may have to adjust to the softer bite of **blackstrap molasses, which contains high amounts of balancing minerals such as calcium, iron, potassium, magnesium, zinc, copper and chromium.** Use it as a sweetener in cakes, pies and cookies. Barbados molasses is sweeter and more syrupy than blackstrap; it is perfect for baking but lacks blackstrap's minerals. **(Note: Diabetics should not use any type of molasses.)**

SWEETENERS TO AVOID

I would avoid any artificial sweetener. Currently Splenda® is being marketed as a viable product. I do not encourage any chemically altered product. Look at the bright yellow wrapper on Splenda®. It says, "Sourced from Sugar." Now let me ask you something; do you consider sugar nutritious? Of course not. I would also not put NutraSweet®, Equal® or any other new product in my body. Why would you want to put additional stress on an already over-worked liver? What about other refined sugars?

Brown sugar is simply refined sugar that is sprayed with molasses to make it appear more whole. **Turbinado sugar** gives the illusion of health, but is just one step away from white sugar. Tubinado is made from 95 percent sucrose (table sugar). It skips only the final filtration stage of sugar refining with little difference in nutritional value.

Corn syrup is found everywhere. It is used in everything from bouillon cubes to spaghetti sauce and even in some "natural" juices. Corn syrup processed from cornstarch is almost as sweet as refined sugar and is absorbed quickly by your blood. Corn-derived sweeteners pose other problems: they often contain high levels of pesticide residues that are genetically modified and are common allergy producers. This is a cheap and plentiful sweetener often used in soft drinks, candy and baked goods. Corn syrup is very similar to refined sugar in composition as well as effect.

Aspartame, which is a common synthetic sweetener, affects the nervous system and brain in a very negative way. Aspartame is made from two proteins, or amino acids, which gives it its super sweetness. Aspartame has many harmful effects: behavior changes in children, headaches, dizziness, epileptic-like seizures, and bulging of the eyes to name a few. Aspartame is an "excitotoxin," a substance that over stimulates neurons and causes them to die suddenly (as though they were excited to death). One of the last steps of aspartame metabolism is formaldehyde. The next time you consume diet soda, think. You are literally embalming yourself.

Sucrose is found in white sugar and maple syrup. Sucrose requires very little digestion and provides instant energy followed by plummeting blood sugar levels. It stresses the entire body system.

Glucose is also called **dextrose**. When combined with sucrose, glucose subjects your blood sugar to the same ups and downs. In whole food form — in starches like beans and whole grain breads, they are also rich in soluble fiber.

Sorbitol, **Mannitol** & **Xylitol** are synthetic sugar alcohols. Although these can cause less of an insulin jump in glucose to sugar, many people suffer gastric distress. You see these listed as ingredients in foods.

Unrefined cane juice. This is sugarcane in crystal form. Nothing more, nothing less. Unrefined cane juice is brown and granulated, contains 85 to 96.5 percent sucrose, and retains all of sugarcane's vitamins, minerals and other nutrients. **Cane juice** has a slightly stronger flavor and less intense sweetness than white sugar.

Crystalline fructose. This refined simple sugar has the same molecular structure as fruit sugar. It's almost twice as sweet as white sugar, yet releases glucose into the bloodstream much more slowly. Extra sugar gets stored in your liver as glycogen instead of continuing to flood your bloodstream.

SUGAR SUBSTITUTION
Amount Indicates the Equivalent of 1 Cup of White Sugar

Sweetener	Amount	Liquid Reduction	Suggested Use
Honey	½ - 2/3 cup	¼ cup	All-purpose
Maple syrup	½ - ¾ cup	¼ cup	Baking & desserts
Maple sugar	½ - 1/3 cup	None	Baking & candies
Barley malt syrup	1 - 1½ cups	½ cup	Breads & Baking
Rice syrup	1 - 1/3 cups	½	Baking & cakes
Date sugar	2/3 cup	None	Breads & baking
Blackstrap molasses	½ cup	¼ cup	Breads & baking
Fruit juice concentrate	1 cup	1/3 cup	All-purpose
Stevia	1 tsp/cup of water	1 cup	Baking

(Note: if you have a serious blood-sugar regulation problem, such as diabetes or hypoglycemia, see your Healthcare Practitioner to determine the type and amount of sweeteners your body can handle.)

It is best to choose food with glycemic indices of 50 — 80. Foods in this range will give us the best chance to minimize exaggerated insulin responses.

GLYCEMIC INDEX

The glycemic index is a measure of food's ability to raise blood glucose to variable degrees. The greater the blood glucose level, the greater the insulin response. Thus, we want to choose food with low glycemic indices. See the Table on page 279. There are many specific benefits of consuming food with low glycemic indices.

1. Blood lipids are reduced in hypertriglyceridemic patients.

2. Insulin secretion is reduced.

3. Overall blood-glucose control improves in insulin-dependent and noninsulin-dependent diabetic subjects.

4. There is a reduction in abnormal blood glucose, insulin and amino-acid levels in patients with cirrhosis.

5. Urinary urea excretion is reduced, presumably by increasing nitrogen trapping by colonic bacteria.

6. Foods with low glycemic indices may enhance satiety.

7. Foods with low glycemic indices may increase athletic performance.

Glycemic Indices of Foods

FOOD	GLYCEMIC INDEX
BREADS	
Rye (crispbread)	95
Rye (whole meal)	89
Rye (whole grain, i.e. pumpernickel)	68
Wheat (white)	100
Wheat (wholemeal)	100
PASTA	
Macaroni (white, boiled 5 min)	64
Spaghetti (brown, boiled 15 min)	61
Spaghetti (white, boiled 15 min)	67
Star pasta (white, boiled 5 min)	54
CEREAL GRAINS	
Barley (pearled)	36
Buckwheat	78
Bulgur	65
Millet	103
Rice (brown)	81
Rice (instant, boiled 1 min)	65
Rice (parboiled, boiled 5 min)	54
Rice (parboiled, boiled 15 min)	68
Rice (polished, boiled 5 min)	58
Rice (polished, boiled 10—25 min)	81

FOOD	GLYCEMIC INDEX
Rye kernels	47
Sweet corn	80
Wheat kernels	63
BREAKFAST CEREALS	
"All Bran"	74
Cornflakes	121
Muesli	96
Porridge oats	89
Puffed rice	132
Puffed wheat	110
Shredded wheat	97
"Weetebix"	108
COOKIES	
Digestive	82
Oatmeal	78
Plain crackers (water biscuits)	100
"Rich Tea"	80
Shortbread cookies	88
ROOT VEGETABLES	
Potato (instant)	120
Potato (mashed)	98
Potato (new/white boiled)	80
Potato (Russet, baked)	118
Potato (sweet)	70
Yam	74
LEGUMES	
Baked beans (canned)	70
Bengal gram dal	12
Butter beans	46
Chickpeas (dried)	47
Chickpeas (canned)	60
Frozen Peas	74
Garden peas (frozen)	65
Green peas (canned)	50
Green peas (dried)	65
Haricot beans (white, dried)	54
Kidney beans (dried)	43
Kidney beans (canned)	74
Lentils (green, dried)	36

FOOD	GLYCEMIC INDEX
Lentils (green, canned)	74
Lentils (red, dried)	38
Pinto beans (dried)	80
Pinto beans (canned)	38
Peanuts	15
Soya beans (dried)	20
Soya beans (canned)	22
FRUIT	
Apple	52
Apple juice	45
Banana	84
Grapes	62
Grapefruit	36
Orange	59
Orange juice	71
Peach	40
Pear	47
Plum	34
Raisins	93
SUGARS	
Fructose	26
Glucose	138
Honey	126
Lactose	57
Maltose	152
Sucrose	83
DAIRY PRODUCTS	
Custard	59
Ice cream	69
Skim milk	46
Whole milk	44
Yogurt	52
SNACK FOODS	
Corn chips	99
Potato chips	77

JUST TELL ME WHAT TO DO!

♦ Avoid all artificial, man-made sweeteners.

♦ Cataplex GTF®, up to nine daily, will minimize sugar cravings. It is a source of chromium.

♦ Reduce your protein amount per serving if you crave sweets after eating them. Consume more small servings of protein to minimize this reaction.

♦ Gymnema®, up to three daily, minimizes the "taste" for sugar.

♦ Focus on local honey as a source of sweetener. The herb, stevia, can be used as a source of sweetener.

♦ Read all labels. Evaporated cane juice, raw sugar, organic crystals — are still sugar.

NOTES_____

_____

_____

_____

_____

_____

_____

_____

Patient Testimony:

"When I first came to see Dr. DeMaria, I had been dealing with minor hot flashes that caused me to break out in sweats during the day. I also had a low thyroid and adult acne. I cut back on my sugar consumption (which was the most difficult) and started to take supplements for my thyroid. The information and care provided by Dr. Bob has improved my life. I have less pain and fewer breakouts on my face."
                                                                Maria Gilmore

Acquiring Your
Normal Weight
Naturally!

Achieving optimal weight levels in our fast-paced lifestyles appears to be eternally elusive. There always seems to be another book or magazine article suggesting that if you eat this food and/or avoid another, your pounds will magically slip away never to return. How many times have you been down that road?

Over my career, I have seen countless people in the same boat, gaining and losing hundreds of pounds. It does not have to get harder as you get chronologically older. I have helped lots of patients lose weight and keep it off. The critical key is to allow the body to heal itself, then watch the pounds melt away naturally. There is no magic bullet, just natural principles that must be followed.

A consistently obese body that does not respond long term to selected food avoidance and portion control, generally, is an unhealthy system. It will not allow the fat to be released because it is being saved for a future time or is so toxic that releasing it results in a self-destructive response. I have had many patients tell me they really watch what they eat, and have been disciplined, but the weight just stays. Is that you? So what is up?

The answer is multi-tiered;

1. A foundation must be built on a solid function hormonal or endocrine system.

2. Detoxification of the cleansing organs.

3. Avoidance of toxic substances.

I am a student of "body watching"; people come in all shapes and sizes. There are visible patterns of fat distribution on the bodies of people who have various organs that are toxic, overloaded and burned out.

Some carry their weight all over the body which suggests thyroid gland distress. These same individuals may have cold hands and feet, high cholesterol and are constipated in addition to some of the other body signals discussed in Chapter Seven on thyroids. They may have small cherry like nodules on their skin, (cherry hemangiomas) suggesting estrogen saturation.

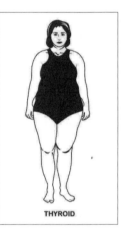

THYROID

Common factors resulting in this scenario include: modern chemicals designed to enhance the production of the food chain and household conveniences that also impair and affect the recipient, i.e., you the consumer. Xenohormones, found in cleaning products, aerosols, lotions, fabrics, paints and many common domestic items, are a part of toxic chain that interferes with normal hormone function. Elevated estrogen levels, whether they are natural or sourced from chemicals, impair thyroid function and congest the liver/gallbladder relationship, resulting in stagnant gallbladder bile flow and congestion.

When the thyroid is hampered in doing its work, you will see an overall-body weight gain. That is why consuming conventionally-sourced animal products, containing synthetic estrogen to "fatten" the animal tissue, has created an enormous challenge for unsuspecting consumers. Clean machines (your body) always work better with the least amount of outside chemicals.

Chlorine in the shower, fluorine in the water and bromine in a pool or hot tub create an extra toxic burden in the body and the liver/gallbladder detoxification system as they compete with iodine receptors. Iodine deficiencies are common in our general dietary food patterns and compound the entire situation. The result is a full figure or thyroid body type.

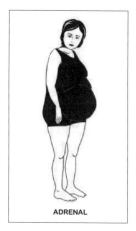

ADRENAL

Stress, whether it is sourced by emotional or physical means, effects an organ in the body called the adrenal gland, as discussed previously. The adrenal gland supplies many critical hormones for our existence; one is called cortisol (cortisone).

When you are under stress, your cortisol levels are up, and you will have a tendency for carbohydrates (cookies, pasta, grain snacks, doughnuts, etc.) to be converted to FAT. What is significant is the fact that "naked sweets" (items that are strictly carbohydrates or refined grain products with "sugar added" and no protein to slow the burn or consumption process down) will result in cortisol being released as a negative feed-back loop to stop the rampage of insulin that is simultaneously being secreted by the pancreas. Patients that are stressed and eating a lot of carbohydrates and stimulants tend to have more of their extra tissue hanging around as a "spare tire" around the waist—the Adrenal Pattern.

Intentional or unaware consumption of toxic food and drink, including artificial sweeteners, taste enhancers, preservatives and

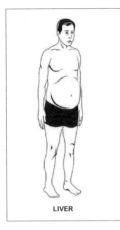

LIVER

even prescription medications, can overload the very important liver-detoxification system. Your liver has many job descriptions. A key function of the liver is to dispose of unwanted and unnecessary substances. Someone that has the huge protruding belly with "humpty-dumpty" bean pole legs will generally have a liver that has expanded and is in a compromised state and currently not working to its full potential. There is fat and fluid hanging over the belt. This particular body type will require real discipline because addictive choices have created this downward spiraling state of health.

Another body shape in a female, at any age after the secondary sexual characteristics appear, that has an accumulation of tissue along the outside aspects of the thighs which can also be combined with an accumulation of tissue in the buttocks. This type can be considered an estrogen-saturation body type and has been classified as the gonadal body. Ovarian malfunction can precipitate this shape. When you do not have enough iodine, your ovaries will not make enough progesterone to balance

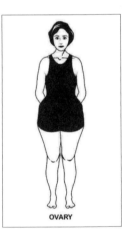

OVARY

the estrogen. I have also noticed that patients who come into the office with "saddle bags," also tend to have liver-congestion issues, which result in unprocessed estrogen. They may have skin eruptions including psoriasis, gallbladder symptoms aggravated by eating fatty or greasy foods, and they may even have high-liver enzymes. It can then be compounded by eating an overload of carbohydrates.

The real challenge is that you can have a combination of body types due to hormonal miscues along with the over-consumption of sweets, lack of exercise and toxic reservoirs.

Let me describe a common picture. A female may have the pattern for the gonadal type with the initial layers of fat being laid down along the thighs, then as the addiction to carbohydrates and sweets becomes ravenous, the additional fat cells are deposited on and along the buttocks. The patient is now contending with a hormonally-initiated addiction to sweets.

An area that is not mentioned is the fact that fat cells can create estrogen. Now this is a double-edged sword for the general population, because today, we are dealing with fake estrogens or xenohormones in unprecedented amounts, which mimic estrogen and stress the liver/gallbladder. Estrogen dominance creates havoc in the body and stresses the liver. You need the liver to process the hormones in the body. The alteration of this loop escalates the fat accumulation dilemma.

An exhausted system, with hormonal depletion, congested toxification of organs, and a general overall state of poor health will not reduce excess fat until it is healthy. If you are struggling and dealing with excessive fat, you need to become healthy and not start another fad diet; otherwise, you will be chasing a state that is not attainable. Now, you cannot get impatient and you do not want to get caught up with the "in moderation" style of eating. No cookies means <u>NO</u> cookies, not even small ones. I don't care how healthy they are. The carbohydrates in them will throw a wrench into their system.

The answer to your problem starts with normalizing the hormonal system in your body. If you do not restart that loop, you will not achieve your optimal health; therefore, you will not lose weight permanently.

The hypothalamus, the chief executive officer, tells the rest of the body what to do. It connects the emotional and physical man. I have seen from experience that it can take anywhere from six months to a year to refuel and restart this hormone loop. If you have had your gallbladder removed it will take longer because the liver has been compromised, and the liver is the hormone recycle depot.

I start with the following protocol food supplement pillar in the hormone foundation by recommending several items to support and restructure the overall hormone system (pituitary, thyroid, adrenal and ovary or testes): Hypothalmex®, 3 daily; Hypothalmus®, 1 daily; Symplex F® for females or Symplex M® for males, 6 daily; 3 Black Currant Seed Oil® capsules, which provide the full spectrum of oils needed as primary ingredients, and Folic Acid B12®, 1 daily. I encourage this support to be used for a minimum of three months. I also suggest that you follow the Page Diet Plan, located in Chapter Twenty, as a template of what to and what not to eat. Avoid any processed food item that has the potential to stress the Phase I and II liver-detoxification process. I would focus on eating cruciferous vegetables: broccoli, cabbage, cauliflower, brussel sprouts and kale. They are best consumed either raw, steamed or sautéed in olive or coconut oil. You should add one Promlamine Iodine® daily if you are focusing on these items. I would recommend that you fill out the Symptom Survey Form and Toxicity Questionnaire in the Appendix to be used as a basis for your foundation, and then fill them out again at the end of the program.

How do you know when you have a proper hormone balance? Well, an objective approach would be to have a mineral-tissue hair analysis and look at the selenium level, which tends to be low with a stressed pituitary. Another marker would be to check your TSH, T3 and T4 before you start the process. A low TSH is often associated with a stressed pituitary. We add Cataplex E®, at a minimum of three daily, to increase the Selenium levels. Also, if you start to see the browning of your skin, this is a signal that your pituitary and liver do not have enough whole-body E. The liver has everything to do with skin lesions. <u>Do not use synthetic vitamin E</u>. Selenium can also be sourced from Cataplex F®, which also has iodine and essential fatty acids.

In our practice we have access to a tool called the Acoustic Cardiogram. It transposes sound energy, made by the valves closing, into a mechanical graph. There are various patterns that can be observed. If we see minimal graph sounds, it indicates that there is a stressed hormonal system. Go to Chapter Fifteen for more details and the location of a practitioner near you.

For one month we have our patients go on a detoxification program focusing on limited foods, with a colon cleanse and green food. Green food is a necessary factor promoting whole body purification. The plan for the month would include protein, gastro fiber, green food and a colon cleanser.

Upon completing the one-month cleanse and having your hormones pointed in the right direction, I assess the major hormonal organ that needs to be focused on. Often there is a combination of one or more. Review Chapters Seven and Eight on Thyroid and Adrenal health. You need to follow the protocols in those chapters.

An important step is to rate the function of the hypothalamus and pituitary. These are not areas in the body that are generally monitored. A periodic hair analysis to monitor the selenium levels and the serum TSH in the thyroid profile is a subtle way to stay on track. Support your system with what you have learned. You may need to stay on the products discussed at the beginning because you may not be able to change your lifestyle and will need to continue to support all your endocrine organs. The supplements I use have never caused any toxic accumulation body signals. I have successfully used them since the early nineteen seventies as a patient and as a Natural Health Doctor.

A couple of points. I generally have to supplement the patient's desire for sweet items. This is a HUGE challenge. Those innocent small morsels have an accumulative affect that tend to settle in the buttocks and thigh region. We really encourage Cataplex GTF®, up to nine daily. GTF has Chromium and helps cool the fire of desiring or craving sugar. Also, Gymnema®, up to three a day, will diminish the taste of sweets. We also use Cholacol®, sourced from bile salts which help take away the passion for sweets.

I would direct you to the Chapter Six on Liver Function and to Chapter Seventeen, the Cleansing Chapter and suggest that you follow the protocols to clean your "machine." This is essential for long-term success on maintaining ideal weight.

For long-term success, you will want to monitor your saliva pH. A patient that is acidic will tend to be more toxic with a greater burden on the whole system which will postpone weight reduction. This could be an issue for some since it is easier to stay in an acidic state, because normal cell metabolism, stress and acid ash foods create an acidic condition.

The glycemic value of food needs to be considered for long-term weight management. I have included a simple glycemic chart available starting on page 279. Focus on foods in the 50 to 80 range (check this). As a side note, even though the foods you consume are in the mid range, do not go overboard and eat a lot. They still have calories. I would avoid the foods in the higher range because they will stimulate insulin release, which is the last fire you want turned on if you want to stay at your ideal weight.

Taking flax oil, at one tablespoon per one hundred pounds of body weight, and avoiding foods that cause inflammation, like sugar, dairy and trans fat, will assist your body in staying at a healthier state. Inflammation that can be detected by having a boggy or spongy wrist, usually suggests that the intestines may be acting like a sieve, with undigested protein particles flowing through the intestines, causing havoc with the immune system and causing the whole body to be on alert, holding on to water to keep the particles in solution. I suggest coconut oil as a medium to cook and as a butter replacement. Coconut oil feeds the hormone circuit and fuels the fire, helping you control the fire that burns the fat tissue.

Trans fat, statistically, when it has been studied and monitored, will actually increase your weight over time. Research on test animals reveals that when compared to other experimental participants will have up to a seven percent increase in weight. That would mean the low fat (trans fat) diet that America has been told is healthy and a way to lose weight is actually wrong.

By following the protocols you have learned throughout the book, your overall system will be working in harmony. Your challenge, as the maestro, is to control the desire for the items that can create craving sugar that releases insulin which crescendos into cortisol release. By far, two of the most significant pieces I can leave with you are—**do not eat sugar and avoid foods that have chemicals added**. Your body has to process each of them and looks at the man-tampered ones as foreign invaders. You will have more challenges managing your weight if you eat synthetic ingredients.

I see so many people today who are extremely overweight, to the point they can hardly walk, and I don't want you to become one or remain as one. If you want to be successful, your focus is to:

- Eat less, eat right...fiber based veggies...and protein
- Avoid trans fat, which in itself causes extra weight

- Drink adequate water
- Avoid all grains and alcohol (including wine)
- Maintain sufficient exercise and sleep patterns
- Avoid stress and over commitments.

Citation: Six Years of Fast-Food Fats Supersizes Monkeys, *New Scientist*, Issue 2556, 17 June 2006, page 21

Patient Testimony:

"I met Dr. Bob in 1984, after I fell on my buttocks on a slippery rock. My mother convinced me to go see Dr. Bob, and he has been monitoring and treating me ever since. Recently, my feet and legs were swelling and I was just miserable, so rather than go to my family physician who would only suggest more medication, I decided to discuss it with Dr. Bob. I made an appointment and brought all of my medications and supplements in and asked him what to do. Dr. Bob was pretty blunt in his approach, but he told me that if I didn't do something now, I wouldn't be around much longer to do anything at all.

Dr. Bob told me to use the Page Fundamental Diet Plan and explained which supplements I should take to get me and my congested liver back on track. Immediately, I started shopping for organic vegetables and meat to eat, doing liver cleanses 2 - 3 times per week, also a colonic and getting lymphatic massages. The change from the food that I was routinely consuming to fundamental organic foods has helped me to lose more than thirty-three pounds in less than twelve weeks. The best part of this story, though, is that I am not hungry. By eating smaller amounts of food, more frequently, I really keep my hunger to a minimum. A lifestyle change like this is normally quite difficult, but I am hopeful that the Page Diet, chiropractic care, lymphatic massages and herbal supplements will help me keep the weight off permanently, while continuing to improve my health."

Terri L. Osborn

THE BODY TYPE QUIZ!

Identifying Your Body Type

Before you take the complete quiz, there are several questions you can ask up front that will quickly tell you if the liver and gallbladder are involved. If the answers to these questions are yes, then you might want to read Chapter Six on the Liver, focus on cleansing and eating items according to the Page Diet.

If you CHECK ANY of the seven points below, you need foods that support the liver. You would do best eating Dr. Bob's ABCs, and initiating the castor-oil pack. You do not need to go through the quiz — you already have your answer. Taking Cholacol ® should be a part of your daily protocol with gallbladder removal.

- ❑ Have you had your gallbladder removed?
- ❑ History of gallstones?
- ❑ Can't lose weight on high-protein diets (e.g., Atkins)?
- ❑ Dislike consuming lots of heavy protein-type foods?
- ❑ Inability to digest fatty or greasy foods, especially at night?
- ❑ History of liver problems?
- ❑ Protruding, distended belly – potbelly?

Directions:
Circle one letter (A, B, C or D) in each question below.
If there is more than one symptom that you are experiencing with a question,
Circle the one that is most prominent.

1. Do you...	A. crave sweets, breads and pasta?
	B. crave salt (pretzels, cheese puffs or salty peanuts) or chocolate?
	C. crave deep-fried foods or potato chips?
	D. crave ice cream, cream cheese, sour cream or milk?
2. Are you...	A. often depressed or feeling hopeless?
	B. a worrier or often anxious and nervous?
	C. irritable, moody, grouchy, in the morning?
	D. moody or irritable at certain times of the month?
3. Do you...	A. feel better on fruits and berries?
	B. need coffee or stimulants to wake up?
	C. experience a tight feeling over your right, lower stomach area or rib cage?
	D. experience constipation during menstruation?
4. Do you have...	A. brittle nails with vertical ridges?
	B. facial hair as a female?
	C. pain/tightness in right shoulder area?
	D. pain in right or left lower back/hip area?
5. Do you have...	A. a weight problem more evenly distributed?
	B. a pendulous abdomen, meaning hanging, sagging and loose?
	C. a protruding abdomen (potbelly)?
	D. excess fat on thighs and hips (saddlebags) and a lower stomach bulge?
6. Do you have...	A. dry skin, especially hands and around elbows?
	B. swollen ankles; socks leave creases on ankles?
	C. flaky skin or dandruff in eyebrows and scalp?
	D. menstrual cyclic hair loss?
7. Do you have...	A. indentations on both sides of your tongue where the tongue meets the teeth?
	B. atrophy (shrinkage) of the thigh muscles with difficulty getting up from a seated position?
	C. dark yellow urine?
	D. hot flashes or history of bad menstruation?

8. Do you have...	A. a loss of hair on the outer third of the eyebrows? B. dizziness when getting up too quickly? C. hot or swollen feet? D. menstrual cyclic brain fog?
9. Do you have...	A. to sleep with socks on at night because of feeling cold? B. chronic inflammation in body? C. headaches or head feels heavy in morning? D. excessive menstrual bleeding?
10. Do you have...	A. puffiness around eyes? B. an unusual feeling of being "out of breath" while climbing stairs? C. skin problems (psoriasis, eczema, brown spots)? D. low sex drive?
11. Do you have... Are you... Do you have...	A. excessive skin sagging under arms? B. twitching under or on top of left eyelid? C. not a morning person, yet feel more awake at night? D. weight gain one week before menstrual period?
12. Do you...	A. have dry hair and hair loss? B. wake up in the middle of the night (2:00-3:00 a.m.)? C. have a deep crevice (deep crease appearance) down the center of tongue and/or a white film on tongue? D. have an upper body which is thinner than your lower body?
13. Do you experience...	A. not being able to maintain curls in your hair after using a curling iron? B. cramps in the calves at night? C. more itching at night? D. water retention at certain times of the month?
14. Do you...	A. become excessively tired in the early evening (7:30-8:00 p.m.) and more awake in the early morning? B. have a more active bladder at night than during the day? C. have a yellow tint in the whites of your eyes? D. have a history of ovarian or breast cysts?
15. Do you have...	A. a lack of get-up-and-go (vitality)? B. calcium issues or deposits – bursitis, tendinitis, kidney stones, heal spurs, early cataracts? C. major moodiness if you skip a meal? D. difficulty losing weight after pregnancy?
16. Do you have...	A. a history of being on low-calorie diets? B. low tolerance for stressful situations, get easily irritable and on edge? C. stiffness and pain more in the right shoulder and right side of neck? D. pain and tightness in one knee, worse during menstrual cycle?

Count up the total of each:

Total A. Thyroid _____ **Total B. Adrenal** _____

Total C. Liver _____ **Total D. Ovary** _____

Weight loss is probably one of the biggest challenges facing our society today. I have seen wonderful results by focusing on improving the hypothalamus and pituitary foundation pillar of hormonal health. I consistently see patients that come into the office who are under stress and have signals of diminished pituitary function. The hair analysis, symptom survey form, and thyroid function tests including the TSH values, have been effective tools helping me monitor and improve body function for my patients. We have had patients, who have never lost weight, see it go away because supplementation and lifestyle modifications create normal function of the brain to body mechanism. The mechanism in the brain is capable of sending the messages that the body needs to function optimally.

NOTES_____

_____

_____

_____

_____

_____

_____

_____

The basis for the information in this Chapter has been taken from *The Seven Principles of Fat Burning: Get Healthy, Lose Weight and Keep It Off,* by Eric E. Berg, D.C.

PART V

CONCLUDING THOUGHTS

25
Finishing
The Puzzle

ay to go! You made it to the beginning of your part of the journey. In other words, you can now end the chapter in your life that has less than optimal hormonal health and create a whole new paradigm. I suggest you evaluate everything you have been exposed to is this book. You should have learned that your body needs to be fed the right, whole foods. It desires to be hydrated with water from a pure source, exercised on a regular basis to maintain structural integrity, have consistent uninterrupted communication from the brain cell to the tissue cell, and the least amount of exposure to outside toxins whether they be from food, drink, water or applications to your outside body.

You have read a lot of new information, and maybe some of the knowledge you have been exposed to has stretched you a bit. You may even be angry. I have a lot of new patients who react that way when they learn the facts. They are angry because they have been given wrong information and allowed their precious organs to be removed. The information you have gleaned will support the structures that you have remaining. I do not want you to think that I am suggesting your body can recreate organs, because it will not. I have had patients think that their gallbladder can grow back. It will not. You need to support the liver if your gallbladder was removed so it will have the proper flow of bile that should trickle at an uninterrupted rate.

I also know that cells can react in a responsive way that has not been totally understood. Cells in your body have the ability to create what the body needs. Not all of this is clearly understood. Science does not have the answer to everything. You may not function to the point where you were pre-surgically, but I have had patients achieve some pretty amazing improvements in body signals by feeding the system the right food and detoxifying the remaining tissue.

An area that I would like to touch on is the fact that if you had surgery, and your symptoms abated, you need to get to the cause of why it happened in the first place. You need to ask yourself, "Why did the organ respond in such a way?" What may seem illusive is actually obvious. Does that make sense? Just because you don't have the symptoms from the organ that was removed, you must ask yourself why did that happen? For example, heavy menstrual flow more than likely suggests estrogen dominance. If you had ablation or a hysterectomy you still have the potential to be in a state of estrogen saturation. If you had your gallbladder removed, and did not change anything else, your liver is still producing thick pasty bile. You need to restore a healthier environment in order for your body to work ultimately.

Do not be misled by well-meaning friends. I am serious about this. I have had many conversations with patients, family and friends who indicate that their associates and acquaintances think they have gone nuts. Friends cannot figure out why you are now eating apples, beets and carrots. These same critics don't think there is anything wrong with having a donut or breakfast pastry. They cannot understand why you are now drinking water instead of "energy drinks." God forbid if you admit that you have decided to avoid liver-stressing alcohol.

You have read many "Just Tell Me What to Do" summaries. I would first start by assessing what you are eating. Focus on eating whole food. I have said that through the whole book. It's a mantra that you will be thankful you chose to live by.

Jan Roberts, a pharmacist and clinical nutritionist in Australia and New Zealand, and author of several books recently mentioned in an article titled, "Addressing Menopause Naturally," in the health magazine, *To Your Health,* March 2007, Issue, that "Women will seek out the products that best support their own efforts and address their core or foundation health. What exactly is core or foundation health, and what are these self-help efforts? First of all, women should know that all of the hormones, neurotransmitters, endorphins and other factors that can reduce menopausal symptoms depend on an adequate supply of vitamins, minerals, amino acids and essential fatty acids. These building blocks come from, or have precursors in, the food and drinks women consume. Unfortunately, most modern diets are unlikely to supply an adequate complement of all those building blocks." That is why it is critical for you to make the appropriate changes necessary to guarantee long-term benefits. You need to seek out the items mentioned in the Page Diet (Chaper Twenty) and Food Transition Guide (Chapter Twenty-One). The food is out there, but you will not find it in a cellophane package or a drive thru , at a fast food or franchise restaurant.

The conventional medical community has not entirely correlated health issues to food yet. I want you to understand that a good portion of your health issues are directly related to what you have done to yourself. It is critical for you to change what you have done to this point. This is a HUGE key to your long-term health.

I would not suggest you go out and start eating a whole bunch of vitamins. Taking vitamins, especially synthetic supplementation, may create more of a challenge than your body can handle.

You do not want to go off your medication without having a consultation with a skilled healthcare provider who has the experience to walk you through restoration steps. You need to focus on feeding your adrenal glands, thyroid gland, ovaries and liver the whole-food vitamins and minerals they need to have to fully function at optimal levels.

I would also, and this will be a challenge but it can be done, avoid soy and wheat products. They both diminish zinc in your body. Also, soy, when you do a study on it, is most often sourced from genetically-modified sources and is processed so much that by the time it gets to your plate it is nearly useless, nutritionally. I know this may be the opposite of what you are hearing. However, for many years everyone was told to use the low-fat, no-fat, trans-fat diet. Where did that get everyone? Soy has a natural affinity to aluminum and has anti-trypsin characteristics. Wheat, with its gluten, causes the villi in the intestine to stick together. This will limit mineral absorption and alter the entire system.

Go to the Food Transition Chart in Chapter Twenty-One and the Page Diet in ChapterTwenty. Review the information and see what you are doing now that would be best to be changed. Do not throw out any food in your house. Use a bit of logic; if you have kids, go slowly.

OK, you are on your way. Don't be anxious, give yourself some time. Slowly start incorporating what you have learned. It will get better, I promise. I have seen it happen so many times before. It is naturally right...

26

Bonus Chapter: Balancing Male Hormones

In my practice I also address the issues that concern male health. I would like to very briefly discuss a few common health nuggets that may help you, as a female, understand what is going on with the men in your life. The balance of male hormones is not as intricate compared to what is going on in a female's body. The primary concern is the cholesterol-originating chart I have included in Chapter Eight on Adrenal Health. Testosterone can be sourced from cholesterol like the other steroid hormones. Review the information I have presented so far about the adrenal glands, liver activity and diet. When men have stress in their daily lives, they will have impaired adrenal function with all the nutrients for cellular function being used to make cortisone to handle the stress and very little left over to make testosterone. Men, in the deficiency mode, lose their desire for sexual intimacy; meaning they can have a decreased libido. I see this commonly on the symptom survey form that I use in my office for patients when I am initiating the whole-body assessment. A lack of sexual desires coincides with a run-down endocrine, or hormone, system. It is as if the spark plugs do not have any fuel to spark. The way the body operates, the nutrients needed to encourage sexual arousal are being used for you to survive.

This following is a common scenario that I see on a very regular basis in my office. The most challenging patient I need to treat and educate is a male between twenty-five and forty-five years old. They still think they have the testosterone and ability of a nineteen-year-old, but in actuality most have the bodies of a fifty-five-year-old instead. They are at the point in their lives where work can be very challenging. There are many financial responsibilities starting to come into reality such as college tuition, larger houses and "toy" payments, i.e., boat, vacation house and club fees.

The weekly recorded diet journal for my male patients is anything but nutritional. Food on the run, along with a night or weekend out with the buddies, does anything but promote a healthy waistline. Cholesterol runs high with this type of lifestyle, the serum readings are near the price of gasoline. Your man just does not feel good.

The pressures of down-sizing at work and fear of the unknown future create the physiology that generates far too many demands. Before he knows it, he has a prescription for blood pressure and cholesterol medication, a "mild" anti-depressant and a new pill to promote an erection. Sound too far out? Not really. I have consultations like this consistently. He needs to eat the foods suggested in Chapter Twenty, The Page Fundamental Diet Plan, as well as follow everything that you are doing. If not, he will suffer with a loss of sexual desire and overall poor health. There was recently an article in the *Wall Street Journal*, Health Matters, entitled, "IS YOUR WIFE PUSHING YOU TO SEE A DOCTOR? READ THIS — AND GO." An interesting comment for you to be aware of in a subtitle: The First to Know, *"Doctors say wives are in a unique position to persuade their husbands to seek medical care. Because erectile function is an important barometer of a man's health."*

I want to describe the physiology of male hormones. I will attempt to keep it simple. Read slowly, I know you will get a better idea of what is going on. Male hormones are called androgens. Androgen is the generic term for any natural or synthetic compound, usually a steroid hormone, that stimulates or controls the development and maintenance of masculine characteristics in vertebrates by binding to androgen receptors. This includes the activity of the accessory male sex organs and development of male secondary sex characteristics. Androgens, which were first discovered in 1936, are also called androgenic hormones or testoids. Androgens are also the original anabolic steroids. They are also the precursor of all estrogens, the female sex hormones. The primary and most well-known androgen is testosterone.

Testosterone is a steroid hormone from the androgen group. Testosterone is primarily secreted in the testes of males and the ovaries of females, although small amounts are secreted by the adrenal glands. It is the principal male sex hormone and an anabolic steroid. In both males and females, it plays key roles in health and well-being. Examples include enhanced libido, energy, immune function and protection against osteoporosis. On average, the adult male body produces about twenty to thirty times the amount of testosterone that an adult female's body does.

Males produce more and females produce less. The human hormone estrogen is produced in greater amounts by females, less so by males. Testosterone causes the appearance of masculine traits, i.e. deepening voice, pubic and facial hairs, muscular build, etc. Like men, women rely on testosterone to maintain libido, bone density and muscle mass throughout their lives. Men rely on estrogens to protect them from prostate cancer.

A subset of androgens, is adrenal androgens which includes any of the steroids synthesized by the adrenal cortex, the outer portion of the adrenal gland. These function as weak steroids, or steroid precursors, and include dehydroepiandrosterone (DHEA). DHEA is a steroid hormone produced from cholesterol in the adrenal cortex, which is the primary precursor of the natural estrogen, androstenedione (Andro): an androgenic steroid, which is produced by the testes, adrenal cortex and ovaries. While androstenediones are converted metabolically to testosterone and other androgens, they are also the parent structure of estrone. Use of androstenedione as an athletic or body-building supplement has been banned by the International Olympic Committee as well as other sporting organizations.

From my continued observation, men would do best to limit their stress, which I know is easier said than done. They also need to minimize the consumption of sugar. Sugar, by far, is a leading cause of poor health. I stopped doing most extra-curricular activities when I was helping to raise our sons. I did not want to burn out my adrenal glands. It is about prioritizing.

Also, as a family, we lived within our budget. Please remember this saying, "your earning power does not ever satisfy your yearning desire." Try to minimize your consumption desire. You won't have to work so hard, which means less stress. Financial concerns are one of the leading causes of divorce in America. One of the purposes of this book was to prevent family issues, including divorce.

I want to share with you a few secret weapons so that you can protect yourself and the men in your life. Men need iodine just like women. I personally supplement myself with up to twelve milligrams of iodine a day. If you have dry eyes, iodine may help. Men who have prostate swelling and/or elevated PSA readings will be pleasantly surprised when those levels go down over time with iodine. I encourage a regular supply of Celtic Sea Salt®, a great source of iodine. I also recommend Prolamine Iodine®; four tablets daily.

Men and women need to check their torso, legs and arms for small, raised, red cherry, bead-like bumps, officially called "cherry hemangiomas." An abundance of these little bumps are a sign to me that there may be estrogen saturation. When men have too much estrogen, they can have prostate issues. A leading factor that increases estrogen in the body is eating conventional versus organic meat. I know that budgets can be limited, however, organic meats are worth saving for.

Both men and women can be impacted by a deficiency of zinc. I generally see a diminished sense of taste and smell in those who need zinc. Eating wheat and soy products will deplete zinc as does sugar and stress. Memory loss, slow healing, white spots on the nails and impaired insulin function can be precipitated by a zinc deficiency. Men need zinc for the prostate to function—this is critical. You may want to get a bottle of the zinc taste test to identify any potential zinc situation.

Men are impacted by blood sugar and adrenal levels which are a part of human hormones. The rules for thyroid also apply for men. Men need to have a balance in all areas to function well, just like women. The natural principles apply to males and females.

Before I give you the final tips, I want you to review this insightful information. Women may have menopause and men can have andropause. This information will give you some insight into the issues males contend with.

Andropause

- Defined as loss of androgen dominance in men
- Caused by functional imbalances in the male hormone pathway wherein free testosterone declines one to two percent yearly while Sex Hormone Binding Globulin gradually elevates compensating for testosterone decline

- Testosterone is made from cholesterol and plays an important role in supporting the thyroid and healthy triglycerides and cholesterol — statin drugs are shown to reduce testosterone

- Symptoms may include: mood swings, depression, pessimism, asthenia, myasthenia, insulin resistance, hypertension, mid-body fat gain, dysglycemia, loss of libido, erectile dysfunction, osteoporosis, prostate/urinary problems, thin dry skin

Andropause vs. Menopause

ANDROPAUSE	MENOPAUSE
➢ Testosterone reduced	➢ Estrogen reduced
➢ Body fat increase	➢ Body fat increase
➢ Biological status decrease	➢ Biological status decrease
➢ Osteoporosis increase	➢ Osteoporosis increase
➢ Cardiovascular dx increase	➢ Cardiovascular dx increase
➢ Prostate cancer increase	➢ Breast Cancer increase

Just Tell me What to Do

- Try for less stress and eat no sugar for optimal testosterone levels.

- Men need to have their Adrenal and Thyroid function up to par to have optimal health.

- Focus on eating protein and veggies versus carbohydrates and sweets which stress adrenal function.

- Have a hair analysis which may show a zinc deficiency and should be treated accordingly. Avoid wheat and soy if your zinc levels are low.

- A quality source of Omega 3 oil of one tablespoon a day per one hundred pounds is a good regime to follow for optimal hormone health.

✝ I use the following protocol personally, and I suggest this to male patients. 3 Hypthalmex®; 1 Hypothalmus PMG®; 3 Black Currant Seed Oil capsules®; 1 Folic Acid B12® and 6 Symplex M® daily for optimal endocrine function. I have the stress of daily living just like other men. This protocol keeps my endocrine system at a level of optimal health.

✝ I stopped consuming alcohol many years ago. I used to have a lot of cherry hemangiomas; I now have one or two. Men need to read Chapter Six on the liver.

✝ Tribulus® is a an herb that can be used to increase the level of testosterone in males and females. This will increase the muscle tone of both of males and females.

✝ You would do best to show this book to the men in your life so they will have a better understanding of women. The puzzle of female hormones is quite intense and needs more than a magic pill for restoration. It is a team effort.

Citation: *Wall Street Journal*, Saturday/Sunday May 12 -13, 2007 Page R9

Concluding
Thoughts

OK, this is it! I pray the information you have learned from these pages has impacted your lives and once again permitted you to become the captain of your own ship. The course that I have plotted for you may not seem easy at first, but trust me, just take baby steps, and do not leave any out and you will be on top of the world without unnecessary surgery. This book is good for the whole family. You will want to talk to both you male and female children and grand children. The game of life is very serious and has a lot of snares that can trap you into a false sense of security. Prescription medication has saved a lot of lives, I am not denying that, but it has also created a lot of permanent injury including premature death. For you to get what you have never received or obtained before, you must now do what you have never done before. Be brave, be the first one in you circle of friends and family to make a difference. It is a matter of life and death. The world is waiting and time is quickly running out.

Be blessed…
Dr. Bob DeMaria

APPENDIX

DIRECTIONS FOR THE SYMPTOM SURVEY FORM

1. Fill in the date, your name, age, surgeries, medications and supplements.

2. Place an "X" in any and all of the boxes by the symptoms that you have on a daily/weekly basis only.

3. Complete the Barnes Thyroid Test at the bottom of the third page. (Even if you do not have a thyroid problem.)

4. Write down everything you eat/drink for one week. List any symptoms you may have at the bottom.

5. Have your blood pressure taken sitting, then immediately standing. Record it.

6. Have your pulse taken sitting, then standing also. Record it.

7. Complete the Iodine Patch Test.

8. You have a couple of options; you can take the form to your natural healthcare provider, and/or make a phone consultation appointment with Dr. Bob or one of his associates, to discuss your state of health. You can go to www.DruglessDoctor.com for details.

NAME: _____ AGE: ____ DATE: _____

SURGERIES: _____

MEDICATIONS: _____

SUPPLEMENTS: _____

(If necessary, attach additional sheet.)

As a result of your consultation, would you prefer to have your personal evaluation report on a cassette or CD? (Circle One)

Instructions: Place an "X" by the symptoms that you notice on a daily or a constant basis.

GROUP ONE

☐ Acid foods upset	☐ Gag easily	☐ Appetite reduced
☒ Get chilled, often	☐ Unable to relax; startles easily	☐ Cold sweats often
☒ "Lump" in throat	☐ Extremities cold, clammy	☐ Fever easily raised
☒ Dry mouth-eyes-nose	☐ Strong light irritates	☐ Neuralgia-like pains
☐ Pulse speeds after meal	☐ Urine amount reduced	☐ Staring, blinks little
☐ Keyed up – fail to calm	☐ Heart pounds after retiring	☐ Sour stomach frequent
☐ Cuts heal slowly	☐ "Nervous" stomach	

GROUP TWO

☐ Joint stiffness after arising	☐ Always seems hungry; feels "lightheaded" often	☐ Constipation, diarrhea alternating
☐ Muscle-leg-toe cramps at night	☐ Digestion rapid	☒ "Slow starter"
☐ Butterfly" stomach, cramps	☐ Vomiting frequent	☐ Get "chilled" infrequently
☐ Eyes or nose watery	☐ Hoarseness frequent	☐ Perspire easily
☐ Eyes blink often	☐ Breathing irregular	☒ Circulation poor. sensitive to cold
☐ Eyelids swollen, puffy	☐ Pulse slow; feels "irregular"	☐ Subject to colds, asthma, bronchitis
☐ Indigestion soon after meals	☐ Gagging reflex slow	
	☐ Difficulty swallowing	

GROUP THREE

☐ Eat when nervous	☐ Heart palpitates if meals missed or delayed	☐ Crave candy or coffee in afternoons
☐ Excessive appetite	☐ Afternoon headaches	☐ Moods of depression - "blues" or melancholy
☒ Hungry between meals	☐ Overeating sweets upsets	☐ Abnormal craving for sweets or snacks
☐ Irritable before meals	☐ Awaken after few hours sleep - hard to get back to sleep	
☐ Get "shaky" if hungry		
☐ Fatigue, eating relieves		
☐ "Lightheaded" if meals delayed		

GROUP FOUR

☒ Hands and feet go to sleepeasily, numbness	☐ Get "drowsy" often	☐ Bruise easily, "black and blue" spots
☐ Sigh frequently, "air hunger"	☐ Swollen ankles - worse at night	☐ Tendency to anemia
☐ Aware of "breathing heavily"	☐ Muscle cramps, worse during exercise; get "charley horses"	☐ "Nose bleeds" frequent
☐ High altitude discomfort	☐ Shortness of breath on exertion	☐ Noises in head, or "ringing in ears"
☐ Opens windows in closed room	☐ Dull pain in chest or radiating into left arm, worse on exertion	☐ Tension under the breastbone, or feeling of "tightness," worse on exertion
☐ Susceptible to colds and fevers		
☐ Afternoon "yawner"		

GROUP FIVE

- ☐ Dizziness
- ☐ Dry skin
- ☐ Burning feet
- ☐ Blurred vision
- ☐ Itching skin and feet
- ☐ Excessive falling hair
- ☐ Frequent skin rashes
- ☐ Bitter, metallic taste in mouth in mornings
- ☐ Bowel movements painful or difficult

- ☐ Worrier, feels insecure
- ☐ Feeling queasy; headache over eyes
- ☐ Greasy foods upset
- ☐ Stools light-colored
- ☐ Skin peels on foot soles
- ☐ Pain between shoulder blades
- ☐ Use laxatives
- ☐ Stools alternate from soft to watery

- ☐ History of gallbladder attacks or gallstones
- ☐ Sneezing attacks
- ☐ Dreaming, nightmare type bad dreams
- ☐ Bad breath (halitosis)
- ☐ Milk products cause distress
- ☐ Sensitive to hot weather
- ☐ Burning or itching anus
- ☐ Crave sweets

GROUP SIX

- ☐ Loss of taste for meat
- ☐ Lower bowel gas several hours after eating
- ☐ Burning stomach sensations, eating relieves

- ☐ Coated tongue
- ☐ Pass large amounts of foul-smelling gas
- ☐ Indigestion ½ - 1 hour after eating; may be up to 3-4 hrs.

- ☐ Mucous colitis or "irritable bowel"
- ☐ Gas shortly after eating
- ☐ Stomach "bloating" after eating

GROUP SEVEN

(A)
- ☐ Insomnia
- ☐ Nervousness
- ☐ Can't gain weight
- ☐ Intolerance to heat
- ☐ Highly emotional
- ☐ Flush easily
- ☐ Night sweats
- ☐ Thin, moist skin
- ☐ Inward trembling
- ☐ Heart palpitates
- ☐ Increased appetite without weight gain
- ☐ Pulse fast at rest
- ☐ Eyelids and face twitch
- ☐ Irritable and restless
- ☐ Can't work under pressure

(B)
- ☐ Increase in weight
- ☐ Decrease in appetite
- ☐ Fatigue easily
- ☐ Ringing in ears
- ☐ Sleepy during day
- ☐ Sensitive to cold
- ☐ Dry or scaly skin
- ☐ Constipation
- ☐ Mental sluggishness
- ☐ Hair coarse, falls out
- ☐ Headaches upon arising wear off during day

- ☐ Slow pulse, below 65
- ☐ Frequency of urination
- ☐ Impaired hearing
- ☐ Reduced initiative

(C)
- ☐ Failing memory
- ☐ Low blood pressure
- ☐ Increased sex drive
- ☐ Headaches, "splitting or rending" type
- ☐ Decreased sugar tolerance

(D)
- ☐ Abnormal thirst
- ☐ Bloating of abdomen
- ☐ Weight gain around hips or waist
- ☐ Sex drive reduced or lacking
- ☐ Tendency to ulcers, colitis
- ☐ Increased sugar tolerance
- ☐ Women: menstrual disorders
- ☐ Young girls: lack of menstrual function

(E)
- ☐ Dizziness
- ☐ Headaches

- ☐ Hot flashes
- ☐ Increased blood pressure
- ☐ Hair growth on face or body (female)
- ☐ Sugar in urine (not diabetes)
- ☐ Masculine tendencies (female)

(F)
- ☐ Weakness, dizziness
- ☐ Chronic fatigue
- ☐ Low blood pressure
- ☐ Nails weak, ridged
- ☐ Tendency to hives
- ☐ Arthritic tendencies
- ☐ Perspiration increase
- ☐ Bowel disorders
- ☐ Poor circulation
- ☐ Swollen ankles
- ☐ Crave salt
- ☐ Brown spots or bronzing of skin
- ☐ Allergies – tendency to asthma
- ☐ Weakness after colds, influenza
- ☐ Exhaustion – muscular and nervous
- ☐ Respiratory disorders

GROUP EIGHT

- ☐ Apprehension
- ☐ Irritability
- ☐ Morbid fears
- ☐ Never seems to get well
- ☐ Forgetfulness
- ☐ Indigestion
- ☐ Poor appetite
- ☐ Craving for sweets
- ☐ Muscular soreness
- ☐ Depression

- ☐ Noise sensitivity
- ☐ Acoustic hallucinations
- ☐ Tendency to cry without reason
- ☐ Hair is coarse and/or thinning
- ☐ Weakness
- ☐ Fatigue
- ☐ Neuralgia
- ☐ Neuritis

- ☐ Nervousness
- ☐ Headache
- ☐ Insomnia
- ☐ Anxiety
- ☐ Anorexia
- ☐ Distraction
- ☐ Confusion
- ☐ Dizziness
- ☐ Instability

FEMALE ONLY

- ☐ Very easily fatigued
- ☐ Premenstrual tension
- ☐ Painful menses
- ☐ Depressed feelings before menstruation
- ☐ Menstruation excessive and prolonged
- ☐ Painful breasts
- ☐ Menstruate too frequently
- ☐ Vaginal discharge
- ☐ Hysterectomy/ovaries removed
- ☐ Menopausal hot flashes
- ☐ Menses scanty or missed
- ☐ Acne, worse at menses
- ☐ Depression of long standing

MALE ONLY

- ☐ Prostate trouble
- ☐ Urination difficult or dribbling
- ☐ Night urination frequent
- ☐ Depression
- ☐ Pain on inside of legs or heels
- ☐ Feeling of incomplete bowel evacuation
- ☐ Lack of energy
- ☐ Migrating aches and pains
- ☐ Tire too easily
- ☐ Avoids activity
- ☐ Leg nervousness at night
- ☐ Diminished sex drive

THYROID PATCH TEST

Purchase a small bottle of Tincture of Iodine and paint a 2" x 2" patch at the crease of your elbow or behind your knee. The iodine patch should be seen for 24 hours. If the iodine patch leaves, it is a sign that your body is utilizing and/or absorbing the iodine. Keep track of the hours that the iodine is visible.

_____ Hours

BARNES PATCH TEST

This test was developed by Dr. Broda Barnes, M.D., and is a measurement of the underarm temperature to determine hypo and hyperthyroid states. The test is conducted by the patient in the a.m. before leaving bed – with the temperature being taken for 10 minutes. The test is invalidated if the patient expends any energy prior to taking the test – getting up for any reason, shaking down the thermometer, etc. It is important that the test be conducted for exactly 10 minutes, making the prior positioning of both the thermometer and a clock important.

PRE-MENSES FEMALES AND MENOPAUSAL FEMALES
Any two days during the month.
FEMALES HAVING MENSTRUAL CYCLES
The 2nd and 3rd day of flow OR any 5 days in a row.
MALES
Any 2 days during the month.

You can do the following test at home to see if you may have a functional low thyroid. Use an oral thermometer or a digital one. When you use a digital one, place the probe under your arm for 5 minutes then turn your machine on; continue on for an additional 5 minutes. When using a regular one, shake down the night before.

DATE: _____ TEMPERATURE: _____

DATE: _____ TEMPERATURE: _____

DATE: _____ TEMPERATURE: _____

DATE: _____ TEMPERATURE: _____

DATE: _____ TEMPERATURE: _____

BP SIT _____ BP STAND _____

PULSE SIT _____ PULSE STAND _____

SALIVA PH _____ BLOOD TYPE _____

Patient's Daily Diet Report

Patient's Name: _____

Dates: From _____ **To** _____

(Be *sure* to list all foods and beverages consumed each day of this Diet Report.)

	1st Day	2nd Day	3rd Day	4th Day	5th Day	6th Day	7th Day
Morning Meal							
Noon Meal							
Evening Meal							
Foods And Beverages Used at Other Times							
SYMPTOMS							

TOXICITY QUESTIONNAIRE

Section I: Symptoms

Rate each of the following based upon your health profile for the past 90 days.

	Circle the corresponding number.
0	Rarely or never experience the symptom
1	Occasionally experience the symptom; Effect is not severe
2	Occasionally experience the symptom; Effect is severe
3	Frequently experience the symptom; Effect is not severe
4	Frequently experience the symptom; Effect is severe

1. DIGESTIVE

a. Nausea and/or vomiting	0	1	2	3	4
b. Diarrhea	0	1	2	3	4
c. Constipation	0	1	2	3	4
d. Bloated feeling	0	1	2	3	4
e. Belching and/or passing gas	0	1	2	3	4
f. Heartburn	0	1	2	3	4

Total: ____

2. EARS

a. Itchy ears	0	1	2	3	4
b. Earaches, ear infections	0	1	2	3	4
c. Drainage from ear	0	1	2	3	4
d. Ringing in ears, hearing loss	0	1	2	3	4

Total: ____

3. EMOTIONS

a. Mood swings	0	1	2	3	4
b. Anxiety, fear, nervousness	0	1	2	3	4
c. Anger, irritability	0	1	2	3	4
d. Depression	0	1	2	3	4
e. Sense of despair	0	1	2	3	4
f. Apathy / lethargy	0	1	2	3	4

Total: ____

4. ENERGY / ACTIVITY

a. Fatigue / sluggishness	0	1	2	3	4
b. Hyperactivity	0	1	2	3	4
c. Restlessness	0	1	2	3	4
d. Insomnia	0	1	2	3	4
e. Startled awake at night	0	1	2	3	4

Total: ____

5. EYES

a. Watery, itchy eyes	0	1	2	3	4
b. Swollen, reddened or sticky eyelids	0	1	2	3	4
c. Dark circles under eyes	0	1	2	3	4
d. Blurred / tunnel vision	0	1	2	3	4

Total: ____

6. HEAD

a. Headaches	0	1	2	3	4
b. Faintness	0	1	2	3	4
c. Dizziness	0	1	2	3	4
d. Pressure	0	1	2	3	4

Total: ____

7. LUNGS

a. Chest congestion	0	1	2	3	4
b. Asthma, Bronchitis	0	1	2	3	4
c. Shortness of breath	0	1	2	3	4
d. Difficulty breathing	0	1	2	3	4

Total: ____

8. MIND

a. Poor memory	0	1	2	3	4
b. Confusion	0	1	2	3	4
c. Poor concentration	0	1	2	3	4
d. Poor coordination	0	1	2	3	4
e. Difficulty making decisions	0	1	2	3	4
f. Stuttering, stammering	0	1	2	3	4
g. Slurred speech	0	1	2	3	4
h. Learning disabilities	0	1	2	3	4

Total: ____

9. MOUTH / THROAT

a. Chronic coughing	0	1	2	3	4
b. Gagging, frequent need to clear throat	0	1	2	3	4
c. Swollen or discolored tongue, gums, lips	0	1	2	3	4
d. Canker sores	0	1	2	3	4
				Total:	

10. NOSE

a. Stuffy nose	0	1	2	3	4
b. Sinus problems	0	1	2	3	4
c. Hay fever	0	1	2	3	4
d. Sneezing attacks	0	1	2	3	4
e. Excessive mucous	0	1	2	3	4
				Total:	

11. SKIN

a. Acne	0	1	2	3	4
b. Hives, rashes, dry skin	0	1	2	3	4
c. Hair loss	0	1	2	3	4
d. Flushing	0	1	2	3	4
e. Excessive sweating	0	1	2	3	4
				Total:	

12. HEART

a. Skipped heartbeats	0	1	2	3	4
b. Rapid heartbeats	0	1	2	3	4
c. Chest pain	0	1	2	3	4
				Total:	

13. JOINTS / MUSCLES

a. Pain or aches in joints	0	1	2	3	4
b. Rheumatoid arthritis	0	1	2	3	4
c. Osteoarthritis	0	1	2	3	4
d. Stiffness, limited movement	0	1	2	3	4
e. Pain, aches in muscles	0	1	2	3	4
f. Recurrent back aches	0	1	2	3	4
g. Feeling of weakness or tiredness	0	1	2	3	4
				Total:	

14. WEIGHT

a. Binge eating / drinking	0	1	2	3	4
b. Craving certain foods	0	1	2	3	4
c. Excessive weight	0	1	2	3	4
d. Compulsive eating	0	1	2	3	4
e. Water retention	0	1	2	3	4
f. Underweight	0	1	2	3	4
				Total:	

15. OTHER

a. Frequent illness	0	1	2	3	4
b. frequent or urgent urination	0	1	2	3	4
c. leaky bladder	0	1	2	3	4
d. genital itch, discharge	0	1	2	3	4
				Total:	

Section I Total: _____

Section II: Risk Of Exposure

Rate each of the following situations based upon your environmental profile for the past 120 days.

16.	Circle the corresponding number for questions 16a – 16f below.

0 Never	**1 Rarely**	**2 Monthly**	**3 Weekly**	**4 Daily**

a. How often are strong chemicals used in your home? (disinfectants, bleaches, oven & drain cleaners, furniture polish, floor wax, window cleaners, etc.)	0 1 2 3 4
b. How often are pesticides used in your home?	0 1 2 3 4
c. How often do you have your home treated for insects?	0 1 2 3 4
d. How often are you exposed to dust, overstuffed furniture, tobacco smoke, mothballs, incense, or varnish in your home or office?	0 1 2 3 4
e. How often are you exposed to nail polish, perfume, hair spray, and other cosmetics?	0 1 2 3 4
f. How often aer you exposed to diesel fumes, exhaust fumes, or gasoline fumes?	0 1 2 3 4
	Total: _____

17.	Circle the corresponding number for questions 17a – 17b below.

0 No	**1 Mild Change**	**2 Moderate Change**	**3 Drastic Change**

a. Have you noticed any negative change in your health since you moved into your home or apartment?	0 1 2 3
b. Have you noticed any negative change in your health since you started your new job?	0 1 2 3
	Total: _____

18.	Answer "Yes" or "No" and circle the corresponding number for questions 18a – 18d below.

	No	Yes
a. Do you have a water purification system in your home?	2	0
b. Do you have any indoor pets?	0	2
c. Do you have an air purification system in your home?	2	0
d. Are you a dentist, painter, farm worker, or construction worker?	0	2
	Total: _____	

Section II Total: _____

GRAND TOTAL (Section I & Section II)	_____

Add up the numbers to arrive at a total for each section, and then add the totals for each section to arrive at the grand total. If any individual section total is 6 or more, or the Grand Total is 40 or more, you may benefit from a Clinical Purification™ program.

Adapted with permission from the author of *Clinical Purification™: A Complete Treatment and Reference Manual*, Dr. Gina L. Nick. Healthcare professionals may obtain complete copies of this book at a professional discount from Standard Process Order Department at 1-800-558-8740. Patients may purchase the book through retail outlets.

Alkaline and Acid Ash Food Groups

A	B	C	E	F	G
Most Alkaline	**Alkaline**	**Lowest Alkaline**	**Lowest Acid**	**Acid**	**Most Acid**
Stevia	Maple syrup, Rice Syrup	Raw Honey, Raw Sugar	Processed Honey, Molasses	White Sugar, Brown Sugar	NutraSweet, Equal, Sweet 'N Low
Lemons, Watermelon, Limes, Grapefruit, Mangoes, Papayas	Dates/Figs, Melons, Grapes, Papaya, Kiwi, Berries, Apples, Pears, Raisins	Oranges, Bananas, Cherries, Pineapple, Peaches, Avacados	Plums, Processed Fruit Juices	Sour Cherries, Rhubarb	Blueberries, Cranberries, Prunes
Asparagus, Onions, Vegetable Juices, Parsley, Raw Spinach, Broccoli, Garlic	Okra, Squash, Green Beans, Beets, Celery, Lettuce, Zucchini, Sweet Potato	Carrots, Tomatoes, Fresh Corn, Mushrooms, Cabbage, Peas, Potato Skins, Olives	Spinach, Kidney Beans, String Beans	Potatoes, Pinto Beans, Navy Beans, Lima Beans	Soybean, Carob
	Almonds	Chestnuts	Pumpkin Seeds, Sunflower Seeds	Pecans, Cashews	Peanuts, Walnuts
Olive Oil	Flax Oil	Canola Oil	Corn Oil		
		Amaranth, Miller, Wild Rice, Quinoa	Sprouted Wheat Bread, Spelt, Brown Rice	White Rice, Corn, Buckwheat, Oats, Rye	Wheat, White Flour, Pastries, Pasta
			Venison, Cold Water Fish	Turkey, Chicken, Lamb	Pork, Beef, Shellfish
	Breast Milk	Goat Milk, Goat Cheese, Whey	Eggs, Butter/Yogurt, Buttermilk, Cottage Cheese	Soy Cheese, Raw Milk, Soy Milk	Cheese, Homogenized Milk, Ice Cream
Lemon Water, Herb Teas	Green Tea	Ginger Tea	Tea	Coffee	Beer, Soft Drinks

RECIPES

Beet & Vegetable Recipes

What's great about beets –

➢ One-half cup of cooked beets is a mere 37 calories.

➢ One-half cup has 17 percent of the Recommended Daily Intake (RDI) for folate, plus vitamin C, potassium, and iron.

➢ Beets give you the cancer-fighting antioxidant beta carotene plus 2 grams of healthy fiber.

➢ They're naturally sweet, but have only 7 grams of sugar per half-cup serving.

Buying tips –

➢ Look for firm beets with smooth skin. Smaller ones are usually more tender than larger ones.

➢ Beets range in color from deep golden yellow to crimson to white.

➢ The lighter the color, the more mellow the flavor. The Chiggia beet is nicknamed "candy cane" because its core is striped with red and white circles

➢ Beets are often sold with their nutritious greens attached. Avoid wilted ones and sauté them like their relative, Swiss chard.

Storing basics –

➢ Cut off the greens, leaving about one inch of stem. Place in a plastic bag and refrigerate for up to two weeks.

Cooking 101 –

➢ Keep the skins on during cooking; this helps retain moisture and nutrients. To remove the skins — and prevent staining, too — rub the cooked beets with a paper towel or run them under cold water while wearing rubber gloves.

> No time to cook? Raw beets can be peeled, grated, and tossed with a light vinaigrette for a quick, healthy salad. Spark up the flavor with grated ginger root or sesame oil.

Did you know…

> It's not an old wife's tale: Urine may turn reddish after you eat beets. This reaction, called beetura, is harmless.

Oven-Roasted Beets

> Rub with olive oil, sprinkle with salt & pepper, and place in a roasting pan. Bake at 375°F for approximately 45 minutes, or until a knife can easily go through the center of the beet. Remove the skins, then slice and serve warm, plain or tossed with butter and vinegar. Or chill the cooked beet slices and layer on top of greens. Dress with vinaigrette, and sprinkle with toasted nuts, and blue or goat cheese.

Shredded Beets with Celery & Dates

Prep: about 10 minutes
Makes about 4 cups or 8 accompaniment servings

1 pound beets, peeled
3 stalks celery, thinly sliced
½ cup pitted, dried dates, chopped
3 tablespoons fresh lemon juice
Salt and coarsely ground black pepper

Cut beets into quarters. In food processor with shredding blade attached, shred beets; transfer to a large bowl. Stir in celery, dates, lemon juice, ¼ teaspoon each salt and pepper. If not serving right away, cover and refrigerate up to 4 hours.

Each Serving: About 50 calories, 1 g protein, 13 g carbohydrate, 0 g total fat, 2 g fiber, 0 mg cholesterol, 110 mg sodium.

Red Cabbage Spaghetti with Golden Raisins

Prep: about 10 minutes
Cook: about 25 minutes
Makes about 8 cups or 6 accompaniment servings

Salt
1 small head red cabbage (about 1½ pounds)
1 tablespoon olive oil
1 small onion, chopped
1 clove garlic, crushed with press
1 cup apple juice
½ cup golden raisins
Pinch ground cloves
8 ounces thin spaghetti (rice pasta)

1. Heat large covered saucepot of cold water and 2 teaspoons salt to boiling over high heat.

2. Meanwhile, discard any tough outer leaves from cabbage. Cut cabbage into quarters; cut core from each quarter. Thinly slice cabbage.

3. In a 12-inch skillet, heat oil over medium heat. Add onion and cook about 8 minutes or until tender, stirring occasionally. Add garlic and cook 1 minute, stirring. Stir in cabbage, apple juice, raisins, clove and ½ teaspoon salt. Cover and cook about 15 minutes or until cabbage is tender, stirring occasionally.

4. About 5 minutes before cabbage is done, add pasta to boiling water and cook as label directs.

5. Reserve ¼ cup pasta cooking water; drain pasta. Stir pasta into cabbage mixture in skillet; add cooking water if mixture seems dry.

Each Serving: About 255 calories, 7 g protein, 50 g carbohydrate, 3 g total fat (0 g saturated), 4 g fiber, 0 mg cholesterol, 275 mg sodium.

Broccoli Gratin

Prep: about 10 minutes
Cook/Broil: about 20 minutes
Makes about 4 cups or 8 accompaniment servings

1 pound broccoli florets
1 pound Yukon Gold potatoes, peeled and cut into 1-inch chunks
2 cups water
Pinch ground nutmeg
¾ cup freshly grated Parmesan cheese (about 2½ ounces)
Salt and coarsely ground black pepper

1. In 4-quart saucepan, place broccoli, potatoes, and water. On high heat, cover and heat until boiling. Then reduce heat to medium-low and cook, covered, 17 – 20 minutes, or until potatoes and broccoli and very tender, stirring once halfway through cooking.

2. Meanwhile, preheat broiler and set oven rack 6 inches from source of heat.

3. Drain vegetables in colander set over large bowl, reserving ¼ cup vegetable cooking liquid. Return vegetables to saucepan. With potato masher or slotted spoon, coarsely mash vegetables adding some reserved cooking liquid if mixture seems dry. Stir in nutmeg, ¼ cup Parmesan, ½ teaspoon salt, and ¼ teaspoon pepper.

4. In shallow, broiler-safe 1- to 1 ½ quart baking dish, spread vegetable mixture; sprinkle with remaining Parmesan. Place dish in oven and broil 2 to 3 minutes or until Parmesan is browned.

Each Serving: About 95 calories, 6 g protein, 13 g carbohydrate, 3 g total fat (2 g saturated), 2 g fiber, 6 mg cholesterol, 305 mg sodium.

Lemon Cilantro Eggplant Dip

Prep: about 10 minutes plus chilling
Roast: about 45 minutes
Makes about 2 cups dip

2 eggplants (1 pound each), each halved lengthwise
4 cloves garlic, unpeeled
3 tablespoons tahini (sesame puree)
3 tablespoons fresh lemon juice
Salt
¼ cup loosely packed fresh cilantro or mint leaves, chopped
Toasted or grilled pita wedges
Carrot and cucumber sticks and red or yellow pepper slices

1. Preheat oven to 450°F. Line 15½" by 10½" jelly-roll pan with nonstick foil (or use regular foil and spray with nonstick cooking spray). Place eggplant halves, skin-sides up, in foiled-lined pan. Wrap garlic in foil and place in pan with eggplants. Roast vegetables 45 to 50 minutes or until eggplants are very tender and skin is shriveled and browned. Unwrap garlic. Cook eggplants and garlic until easy to handle.

2. When cool, scoop eggplants' flesh into food processor with knife blade attached. Squeeze out garlic pulp from each clove and add to food processor with tahini, lemon juice, and ¾ teaspoon salt; pulse to coarsely chop. Spoon dip into serving bowl; stir in cilantro. Cover and refrigerate at least 2 hours. Serve dip with pita and vegetables.

Each tablespoon: About 10 calories, 0 g protein, 2 g carbohydrate, 0 g total fat, 1 g fiber, 0 mg cholesterol, 55 mg sodium.

Sesame Ginger Brussels Sprouts

Prep: about 15 minutes
Cook: about 15 minutes
Makes about 4 cups or 8 accompaniment servings

2 containers (10 ounces each) Brussels sprouts
2 tablespoons Worcestershire sauce
2 teaspoons grated, peeled fresh ginger
1 teaspoon Asian sesame oil
1 tablespoon olive oil
1 large onion (about 12 ounces), cut in half and thinly sliced
2 tablespoons water

1. Trim stems and any yellow leaves from Brussels sprouts. Cut each sprout lengthwise into quarters. In cup, stir together soy sauce, grated ginger and sesame oil.

2. Meanwhile, in nonstick 12-inch skillet, heat olive oil over medium heat until hot. Add onion and cook about 5 minutes or until it begins to soften, stirring occasionally.

3. Increase heat to medium-high; add Brussels sprouts an water; cover and cook about 5 minutes or until sprouts are beginning to soften and brown, stirring once. Remove cover from skillet and cook about 5 minutes longer or until sprouts are tender-crisp, stirring frequently. Remove skillet from heat; stir in soy sauce mixture.

Each Serving: About 65 calories, 3 g protein, 10 g carbohydrate, 3 g total fat (0 g saturated), 3 g fiber, 0 mg cholesterol, 165 mg sodium.

Strawberry Spinach Salad

Prep: about 5 minutes
Makes about 12 cups or 6 accompaniment servings

1 pound strawberries, hulled and sliced
2 tablespoons plus 1 teaspoon white balsamic vinegar
1 tablespoon olive oil
Salt and coarsely ground black pepper
2 bags (5 go 6 ounces each) baby spinach
3 ounces goat cheese, such as Montrachet, crumbled (¾ cup)
¼ cup sliced almonds, toasted (see note)

1. In blender, puree ¾ cup strawberries with vinegar, olive oil, ¼ teaspoon salt, and 1/8 teaspoon pepper. Transfer vinaigrette to large serving bowl.

2. Add spinach and remaining strawberries to bowl and toss to coat with dressing. Crumble goat cheese over top of salad and sprinkle with toasted almonds.

Each Serving: About 115 calories, 6 g protein, 7 g carbohydrate, 8 g total fat (3 g saturated), 7 g fiber, 7 mg cholesterol, 215 mg sodium.

Editor's Note: To toast sliced almonds, place in small skillet and cook over medium heat 2 to 3 minutes or until golden, stirring occasionally. Transfer to a plate to cool.

Make It Quick

1. Oven-Roasted Brussels Sprouts

Trim and halve Brussels sprouts from two 10-ounce containers; toss in jelly-roll pan with 1 tablespoon olive oil. Roast in preheated 450°F oven 20 to 25 minutes or until tender and browned, stirring once or twice. Toss with 2 tablespoons seasoned rice vinegar and pepper to taste. Serves 4.

Each Serving: About 95 calories, 4 g protein, 14 g carbohydrate, 4 g total fat (0.8 g saturated), 5 g fiber, 0 mg cholesterol, 295 mg sodium.

2. Basil & Balsamic Beets

In 13" by 9" roasting pan, toss 2 pounds beets with 1 tablespoon olive oil. Roast in preheated 450°F oven 1 hour or until tender. Cool beets; peel and discard skins. Dice beets; toss with 2 tablespoons each chopped fresh basil and balsamic vinegar, 1 tablespoon honey, and ¼ teaspoon salt. Serves 4.

Each Serving: About 115 calories, 2 g protein, 19 g carbohydrate, 4 g total fat (0.5 g saturated), 4 g fiber, 0 mg cholesterol, 260 mg sodium.

3. Grilled Eggplant with Feta and Fresh Mint

Cut one large eggplant (about 1 ½ pounds) into ½-inch thick slices; brush each slice with 2 tablespoons olive oil. Place on hot, ridged grill pan over medium-high heat; cook eggplant slices 4 to 5 minutes per side or until tender. Transfer to platter. Sprinkle with ¼ cup feta cheese, 2 tablespoons chopped fresh mint, and a drizzle of fresh lemon juice. Garnish with lemon wedges. Serves 4.

Each Serving: About 105 calories, 3 g protein, 9 g carbohydrate, 7 g total fat (2 g saturated), 4 g fiber, 8 mg cholesterol, 110 mg sodium.

CITATIONS

Why Am I Always Tired, by Anne Louise Gittleman Chapter Eleven

The Relaxation and Stress Reduction Workbook, by Martha Davis Ph.D., Elizabeth, MSW, and Mathew M. Kay, Ph.D.

Your Liver Your Life Line, by Jack Tips Ph.D.

Adrenal Fatigue, by James Wilson, Ph.D., ND

Setting Things Straight, by John Maderia, D.C.

The 7 Principles of Fat Burning, by Eric Berg D.C.

The Ultimate Healing System, by Don Lepore N.D.

Fats That Heal and Fats That Kill, by Udo Erasmus

Dr. Bob's Trans Fat Survival Guide, by Robert DeMaria, D. C., N.H.D.

Dr. Bob's Guide to Stop ADHD in 18 Days, by Robert DeMaria, D.C., N.H.D.

The Answer to Cancer, by Hari Sharma, M.D. and Rama K. Mishra, G.A.M.S.

PRODUCT INQUIRY

There are many companies that create products that are excellent. I have personally used and have recommended the items I have mentioned in the book with consistent success. You may in fact have a source of items that have produced the health restoration results you have used to help yourself and or others if you are a healthcare provider. I would encourage you to use what you have found successful but, if you are like so many that come into my office with boxes and bags of partially used bottles and have experienced minimal or no improvement maybe it is time to seek other options.

It has been reported that one half of the public in the United States consume some type of supplementation on a regular basis. According to a recent survey of 1,000 supplements conducted by ConsumerLabs.com, a product certification company, one of four supplements has quality problems such as contamination or a failure to include ingredients listed on the label. The companies and items I have suggested have a long track record of quality products.

If you are not familiar with the items I have discussed you can go to the Web pages of the manufacturers I have suggested and request a provider in your area. I have many direct referrals from these companies because the products discussed are of the highest quality and patients are seeking answers for their health concerns. The material used for other procedures including Nitrazine Paper, Flannel, Castor Oil, etc. can be obtained from a local health-food store

If you are unable to locate the products you can call 1-888-5672 or email druglesscare@aol.com or search www.DruglessDoctor.com.

I have used the following nutritional product lines:
- ➤ Standard Process Labs and Medi Herbs
- ➤ Omega Nutrition
- ➤ The Grain And Salt Company

Diet-Supplement Rules Tighten, Saturday-Sunday June 23-24, 2007, the *Wall Street Journal*, Page A3, Jane Zhang

CONSULTATIONS AND SERVICES

I frequently am asked to answer questions in regards to conditions individuals are not receiving answers for. I would suggest you exhaust your local healthcare provider community. If you are not able to receive answers then you can have a phone consultation with me or one of my associates. We also have patients travel to our clinic. You can visit my web page at www.DruglessDoctor.com for details. Procedures including hair analysis, saliva testing and other screens can be completed long distance. You would follow the same procedure as you would for a consultation, since these services would need to be sent to the appropriate lab.

SEMINARS-WORKSHOPS-WELLNESS EVENTS
BUSINESSES-CHURCHES-ORGANIZATIONS

I am available on a limited basis to travel to your location. There is time schedule and attendance minimums required. I generally need to schedule six months to one year out, so if you are thinking about having a special event please contact us early, 1-888-922-5672 or email druglesscare@aol.com.

Index

A

Acid ash diet
  and osteoporosis 107
Acoustic Cardiogram 183
Adrenal
  body type 285
  fatigue
    factors leading to 94
    checklist 93
  glands 13, 89-99
    functions of 91
Alkaline/Acidic Food Chart 323
Amasake 273
Androgenic hormones 305
Androgens 305
Andropause 307
Antidepressants 225
Aspartame® 272, 276

B

Ball exercise 128
Barley malt syrup 273
Blackstrap molasses 275
Blood Pressure 176
Body types 285-286
  identifying 293
  quiz 293
Bone loss 106
Brain cell to tissue cell
  connection 122
Breast cancer
  underlying issues of 193
Brown rice syrup 272
Brown sugar 276

C

Calcium 108

Castor oil 202
  common ailments it can
    remedy 204
  rubbed into the skin 204
  pack 201, 204
    benefits of 206
Cat stretch 128
Celtic Sea Salt® 82
Cherry hemangiomas 307, 309
  estrogen saturation 284
Cholesterol
  and cortisone 254
  and fats 253
  chart 90
  functions in the body 254
  HDL & LDL 256
Cleansing protocals 70, 201-218
Clinical Testing 179
Coffee enema 72, 213
  procedure 215
Cold sores 108
Colon 61
Colonic 70
  irrigation 207
Concentrated fruit juice
  as a sweetener 275
Corn syrup 276
Crystalline fructose 277

D

Date sugar 275
Dextrose 277
DHEA 53, 306
  deficiency, sypmtoms of 53
  excess, symptoms of 54
Digestive aides 228
Door Jam Push-Up 127

E

Endocrine system
  glands of the 13
  processes regulated by 12
Estrogen 29-42
  and soy 219
  and the liver 29
  body type 286
  breast cancer 193
  cherry hemangiomas 284
  deficiency, symptoms of 37
  dominance 67
  excess, metabolic problems
    of 38
  excess, symptoms of 38
  high levels 46, 48-49, 85, 195
  hot flashes 143
  in men, prostate cancer
    protection 305
  know functions of 37
  menopause 308
  saturation 95
  source of 13
  therapy
  three main 36
  to slow osteoporosis 106
Exercise 127-128, 165-170
  benefits of 165
  options 166
  sore muscles, how to avoid
    168

F

Fat
  facts about 251-270
  phobia 79
Food Transition Guide 247-250
  charts I - IV 248-249
Fructose 274
Fruitsource® 273

G

Gallbladder/Liver Flush 207, 209

Glucose 277
Glycemic index 271, 278
  of foods 279

H

HDL cholesterol 256
Herpes 109
Honey 274
Hormonal-based conditions 133
Hormone Replacement Therapy
  (HRT) 20
Hormones 11-28, 53-57
  and fat 251
  androgenic 92
  bio-identical 198
  soy sourced 19
  feel-good 165
  female
    estrogen 36
  male 303
  sex 13, 25
  steroid 32, 44-45
  synthetic 18, 22, 24
  thyroid 38, 80-81
Hot flashes 112, 141-154
  causes of 143
  help for 147
  symptoms of 143
  triggers 147
Hydrogenated Oil 257
Hypothalamus 13, 15

I

Iodine phobia 82

L

LDL cholesterol 256
  high levels from trans fat
  complications from 261
Leg Blood Pressure 177

Liver 29, 67-75
  body type 286
  flush, reasons for 71
Liver/gallbladder flush 71, 207
Low-fat/no-fat diet fad 259
Lymph nodes 57
  swollen 58
Lymphatic
  cancer 57, 63
  drainage massage 61
  system 57-65

M

Male hormones 303-310
Maltose 274
Mannitol 277
Maple syrup 274
Medication
  how to get off of 225-230
Mineral Tissue Analysis 183
Monounsaturated fats 252

N

Nervous system 122

O

Osteoclast 102
Osteoporosis 101
  estrogen therapy 106
  factors leading to 107
  medications 102
Ovaries 13
Ovary body type 286

P

Page Fundamental Diet Plan
  233-245
Palpation 179
Pancreas islets 13
Parathyroid 13

Partially-hydrogenated oil 257
Patient's Daily Diet Report 319
Pineal gland 13
Pituitary gland 13
Poison Ivy 119
Polyunsaturated fat molecules
  253
Premarin 20
  problems with 21
PremPro 23
Progesterone 16, 43-52
  source of 13
  synthetic 23
Progestins
  problems with 23
Provera 23

R

Recipes 324-331

S

Saliva
  tests 172-174
Salt phobia 82
Saturated fats 252
Soda
  and osteoporosis 107
Sorbitol 277
Sore muscles
  from exercise 168
Soy
  high aluminum 198
  hot flashes 141
Splenda® 271
Steroid hormone 305
Stevia 273
Stress
  and osteoporsis 107

Structural Restoration
  steps to 115
Subluxation 125
  symptoms of 128
Sucrose 277
Sugar 271
  and osteoporosis 107
  fake 271
  high insulin levels 82
  substitution equivalents 278
Supplements
  calcium lactate 221
  herbs 223
  iodine 222
  minerals 221
  multiple 220
  organ support tissue 222
  protein 221
  soy and bio-identical 223
Sweeteners
  natural 272
Symptom survey 315
Synthetic hormones
  problem with 18

T

Testoids 305
Testosterone 305
  deficiency body signals 55
  excess body signals 55
  in females 54
Tests
  to evaluate your health 171
Thyroid 13, 77, 87
  body type 284
  iodine 79
  medication 227
  symptoms of low TSH 83
Thyroid Stimulating Hormone
  (TSH) 81
Toxicity questionnaire 320

Trans fat 257
  0 grams loophole 264
  and ADHD 264
  leading cause of health
    problems 263
TSH 81
Twin Scales 178

U

Unhealthy Patterns
  reversing 189-200
Unrefined cane juice 277

V

Vertebral column 122
Vitamin B deficiency syndrome
  33
Vitamin D 109

W

Water
  how much to drink 60
Weight
  achieving a normal 283-296
Whole fruit
  as a sweetener 274

X

Xenohormone
  exposure, disorders related
    to 40
  exposure, steps to avoid 40
  sources of 39
X-ray Assessment 185
Xylitol 277

Z

Zinc
  deficiency 195, 307
  test 172

Dr. Bob's Guide to Stop ADHD in 18 Days
A Drugless Family Guide to Optimal Health

Dr. Robert DeMaria
Phone: 440.323.3841

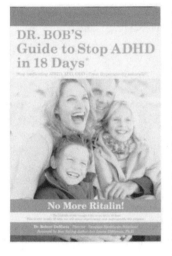

About the Book: SEE IF YOU CAN PASS THE ADHD TEST ON PAGE 8. Anyone can successfully overcome ADHD and Hyperactivity without drugs. This book details how to get your children and family off medications and detrimental junk foods filled with trans-fatty acids, dairy products, sugar and preservatives, so that they can have optimal, natural health. This is a simple, effective step by step plan that includes adding FLAX OIL, modifying your diet and vitamin/ mineral intake. The protocol will improve your nervous system function; help you overcome behavioral and learning problems. It will improve insomnia, mood swings and irritability. The result will be your body healing itself naturally. Participants in the pilot program saw improvement in only 18 days. NATURALLY!!!

About the Author: Dr. Robert DeMaria has been a drugless healthcare provider for over 30 years. He has successfully treated thousands of chronic, difficult cases with the clinical evidence described in Stop ADHD. He has a bachelor's degree in Human Biology; **he graduated the valedictorian of his class** and is currently a practicing DC and consulting NHD. Dr. DeMaria applies his experience daily to help patients without drugs. He teaches, lectures, and has his own television program.

An order form for this book and many other items is included..

"Dr. Bob's Trans Fat Survival Guide: Why No Fat, Low Fat, Trans Fat is KILLING YOU!!"

Dr. Robert DeMaria
Phone: 440.323.3841

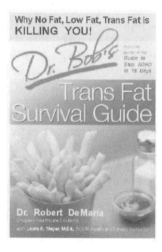

About the Book: This book explains the dangers of trans fat, commonly called hydrogenated and partially hydrogenated fat, as well as how to recognize them in every day foods by properly reading nutritional labels. Along with trans fat, you will learn the different types of fats, which ones are beneficial, and which ones should be used for cooking, baking or eating. Not to leave the reader hanging with questions on how to eliminate dangerous fats and take on a healthier approach to life, there are several sections dealing with how to make those changes, transitioning healthier foods into their eating plan. This book will encourage and empower you to make better choices and learn to live an optimal and healthy life.

About the Author: Dr. Robert DeMaria has been a drugless healthcare provider for over 30 years. He has successfully treated thousands of chronic, difficult cases with the clinical evidence detailed in the Trans Fat Guide. He has a bachelor's degree in Human Biology; **he graduated the valedictorian of his class** a practicing DC and consulting NHD. Dr. DeMaria applies his experience daily to help patients without drugs. He teaches, lectures, and has his own television program.

About the Author: Laura Meyer, M. Ed. and certified personal trainer was a high school English teacher for 13 years. She also holds a Health and Fitness Instructor certification from the American College of Sports Medicine. She is committed to healthy living and encourages her clients as they make healthy lifestyle changes.

An order form for this book and many other items is included.

Dr. Bob's Guide to Optimal Health

A God-Inspired, Biblically-Based 12 Month Devotional
to Natural Health Restoration

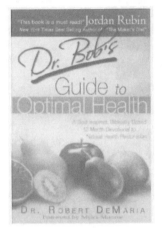

The Guide to Optimal Health is a Spirit of the Lord inspired collection of over 300 natural health tips. It has been designed to slowly transform the reader's life to one of the finest health. Experience in treating patients suggests that it may take twenty-one days to create a new habit pattern. The first of 18 different patterns discussed is water. There are twenty-one daily natural health tips and associated Bible verses focusing on water. There is a daily **Natural Prescription for Health.** At the end of the Guide there are several reference tables including a Food Combining Chart, Glycemic Index, a Good and Not So Good Sweeteners, a pH Chart, and a Transition Food Guide. The material you will learn will empower you to make choices that will have eternal impact on you, your family and friends.

About the author: Dr. Bob DeMaria is an experienced, natural healthcare provider. He has focused his career on helping patients with drugless therapeutic protocols. Dr. Bob has a degree in Human Biology, specialties in Spinal Engineering and Natural Orthopedic Treatment. . **He graduated cum laude and the valedictorian of his class.** He practices clinically as a Chiropractor (DC). He consults worldwide as a Natural Health Doctor (NHD).

Dr. Bob co-hosts a TV program along with his wife of 30 years, Deb. He has been a college instructor, team physician, business health consultant and post-graduate trainer in the legal and health fields. He has written two other books, *"Dr. Bob's Guide to Stop ADHD in 18 Days"*, and *"Dr. Bob's Trans Fat Survival Guide"*. He is an international speaker, has served as an expert witness, and has been in an active practice since 1978. He gave his life to the Lord in 1987. He and his wife appreciate the prayers of all who read this devotional guide to optimal health. A portion of the proceeds from this Devotional will be used to financially support Bethany Blessing Ministry.

An order form for this book and many other items is included.

Dr. Bob's TOP 10

WORKSHOPS TO WELLNESS

VOLUMES I & II

Enjoy listening to Dr. Bob's timely nuggets at your leisure in the comfort of your own home, downloaded on your Ipod, or in your vehicle. Dr. Bob's "Top 10 Workshops to Wellness" are professionally, quality recorded audio CD's including the BEST of the actual weekly workshops that Dr. Bob gives to his patients in the clinic. You may not be there in person, but you can enjoy the current information any time you want. There is also a printable outline available on each CD. The outline can be accessed from your desktop through the search link on "my computer". The timely topics include:

VOL. I

1. Lose Weight Without Dieting
2. Helping Depression Without Drugs
3. Tips to Optimal Health...Naturally
4. Why am I Always Tired
5. Helping Allergies Naturally
6. The Drugless Approach to Hormone Replacement Therapy
7. Helping High Blood Pressure Naturally
8. The Breast Cancer Pattern
9. Improving Your Sexual Desire Naturally
10. Lower Your Cholesterol Without Drugs.

VOL. II

1. Helping Fibromyalgia Naturally
2. 16 Turbo Charged Health Tips
3. Herbs for Life
4. Understanding Thyroid Function
5. Detoxification
6. Let Food Be Your Medicine and Medicine Be Your Food
7. Zinc: The Necessary Nutrient
8. Nuts to Soy... the Hidden Truth
9. ADHD-Depression-Alzheimer's-Memory Loss
10. Controlling Asthma without Medication